How to Attract Women

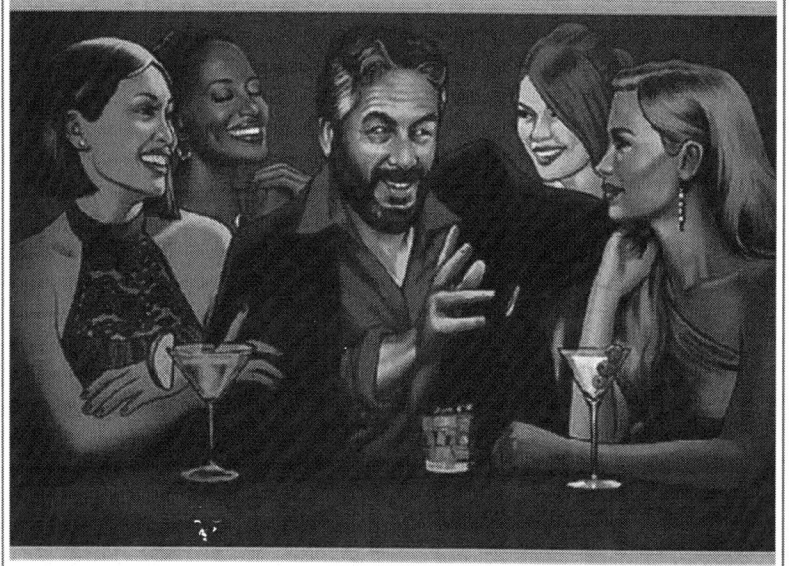

The Irresistible Humor and
Body Language Secrets

Leonardo Bustos

HOW TO ATTRACT WOMEN
THE IRRESISTIBLE HUMOR AND BODY LANGUAGE SECRETS

Written and Narrated By

Leonardo Bustos

****

If you want to attract more women and make them want you, I will take you through a step by step formula that will easily help you to develop the attractive humor skills and alpha male body language habits that women are subconsciously attracted to at a primal level.

You will discover how fun and exciting it is to confidently approach practically any woman, anytime, anywhere and instantly have a fun and humorous connection with her. I'll share with you a guaranteed foolproof method that has never failed me in over a hundred times I've used it...

Men are aroused more by visual cues. A man looks at a woman searching for sexual stimuli like a jeweler looks for perfection in a flawless gem. Visual cues convey information about a woman's health, fertility, and youth.

Women are aroused more by psychological cues. A woman looks at a man much like a detective would a suspected criminal who is about to commit another crime. The visual cues a woman looks for are status, resources, commitment, kindness, stability, and humor.

Just as you are attracted to a beautiful face, ass, and breasts, so are women attracted to "male cleavage," or the attractor factors that include attractive humor and alpha body language. I'm going to show you how to develop those psychological cues that women can't help but be attracted.

With a little practice, you'll start to notice that women will begin to smile at you more when you stimulate the emotional part of their brains that make them laugh. You'll especially notice how they will start engaging you more in a playful manner and will then want to start spending more time with you.

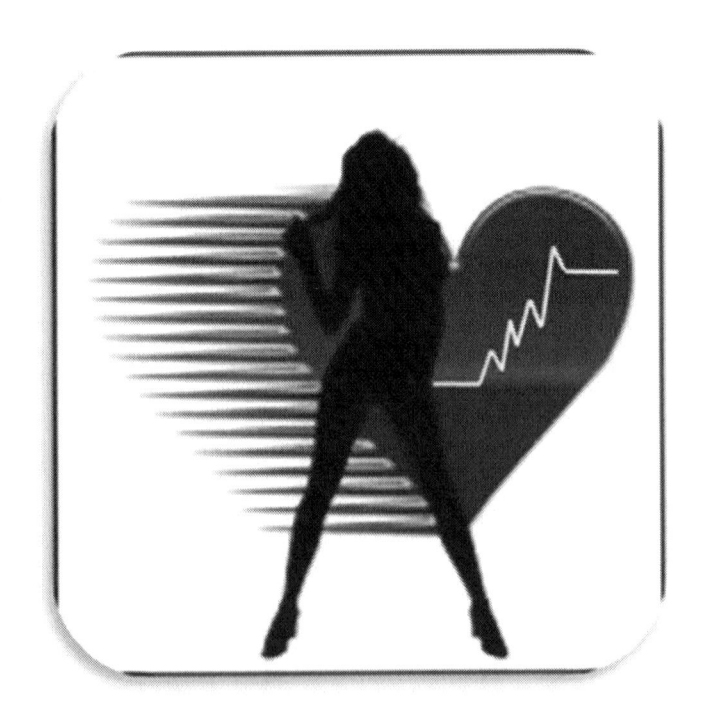

Sign up for free dating advice and videos on how to attract women at

www.TheCompanionator.com

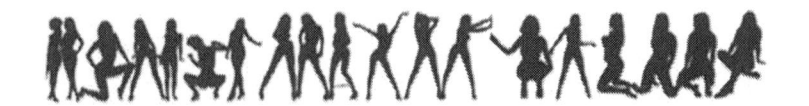

HOW TO ATTRACT WOMEN:

1. Don't be a Dick

2. Don't be a Pussy

Written and narrated by Leonardo Bustos

Copyright 2015 by Amorado Cloud Productions

Audiobooks thanks you for your purchase, and you can find more books written and narrated by Leonardo by going to his website,

"Come on man, you gotta' do more than that…"

What's that, you want more?

There's more…

INTRODUCTION:

HOW TO ATTRACT WOMEN WITH HUMOR – THE DEMONSTRATION

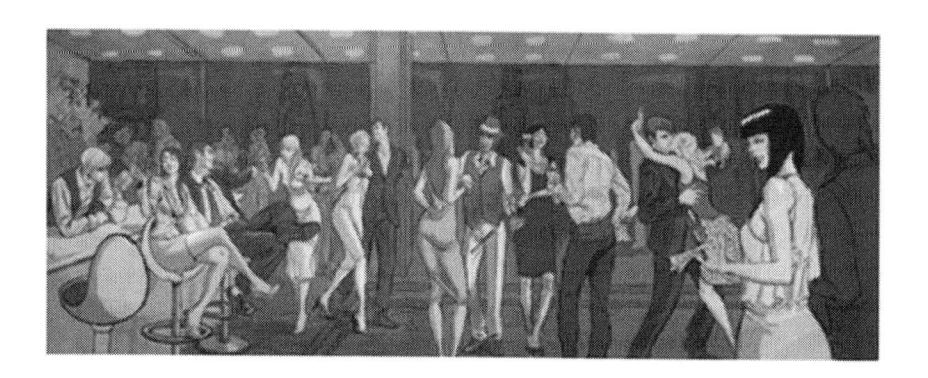

Here's how a professional does it – imagine this scene…

I arrive at the epic singles party of the year.

A few lingerie models, a couple of flexible yoga instructors, and other attractive females of various occupations have arrived. Even a top female MMA fighter is supposed to show up. It's taking place at a fancy hotel in Newport Beach and a wealthy friend I've known for years invited me. He warned me with a raised eyebrow and a grin "Remember our Cub Scout motto - be prepared."

I enter the softly lit club with great anticipation. The sensual sounds of a jazz quartet welcome me. The music is blending in with muffled conversations highlighted by an occasional outburst of laughter. Assorted eye candy adorns the room in the form of shapely breathtaking babes in revealing outfits.

The sexual tension in the air permeates my senses. I can't decide if the sensation comes from the vision of attractive women blended with their subtle notes of perfume wafting through the air, or the invisible scent from their pheromones of pent up desires. I'm guessing both.

Drinks are flowing freely and the place is starting to loosen up. "The games have officially begun," I tell myself with a smile.

The object of "the game" is to apply your social and dating skills in a hunt to locate and hook up with a mystery target who is yet to be identified somewhere in the crowd. The reward is an intoxicating sensation of your mental and physical pleasure centers lit up like flashing lights and ringing bells when you hit a jackpot on a slot machine. The trophy you'll get to take home is the yet unidentified mark.

Matt McConaughey would be a high value target for the women if he showed up tonight, but since it's highly unlikely he won't, I'm going to borrow his character. No one is going to know and I'm sure he won't care.

I glance at myself as I slowly pass by a mirror and with the sexiest, most devilish grin I own; I say under my breath, "All right, all right all right... wherever I am, that's the place to be —now it's Showtime!"

I slowly enter the crowded main room with absolute confidence like a rock star walking on stage. I feel in harmony with my body language, attitude, and masculine energy. On the drive over, I mentally rehearsed my playlist and already imagined myself giving a successful performance ending with an encore.

With my chin slightly up, I scan the room as if I'm about to select from the section of a catalogue featuring a bunch of adoring groupies. The lucky winner in tonight's crowd will be the first worthy woman to show me an i-o-i, or indication of interest.

I spot a gorgeous Latina giving me the eye and I employ the 3-second rule. I start my 3-second approach because I can tell she's open to my advance by her welcoming body language, facial expression, and eye contact.

It looks like God himself just finished spray-painting on her a revealing, form fitting, sexy red dress that leaves very little to the imagination. She pretends to ignore the effect her visual display has on the plentiful number of onlookers, male and female. Imagine Sofia Vergara's younger sister.

The chilled room causes her high beams to attract more eyeballs than moths fluttering to matching porch lights on a dark night, but I pretend not to notice them.

My first thought is to rescue and release her ample breasts from the confining captivity of their tightly bound constraints. Only then, can I comfort and console them with tender caresses and kisses, because after all, I am that sensitive, thoughtful type of guy…

She is stunning. Her full moist red lips perfectly match the color of her dress. Her lingering seductive eyes cause in me a primal arousal that desires fulfillment, but I temporarily put that thought on hold because I can't be distracted from my mission.

I make my move. I tell myself to stay focused because this is where most amateurs typically fail. I'm not an amateur.

She's chatting it up with a few girlfriends as she watches me approach. Then she flashes me the smile. All of a sudden, it feels like I'm onstage under a spotlight.

A hush comes over the room and I imagine everyone is now watching us out of the corners of their eyes while trying to listen inconspicuously. They are waiting and wanting to see what's going to happen next because they know I'm about to make my move.

I slowly stroll over and stand beside her as I look out at the crowd. I can feel her gaze and tension build slightly as I wait for just the right moment to ask her casually …

"So, do you know when the uh…, the attractive women are going to get here?"

Suddenly, as if the DJ loudly scratched the needle across a record, it seems like everything reverts to normal. The sounds return and our imagined audience goes back to what they were doing.

"Excuse me?" She says, as she looks me up and down in disbelief.

I keep a straight face as I calmly move from against the wall to face her at a 45% angle, and give her the eye triangle technique. I slowly look at her left eye, over to her right, then down to her luscious lips where I allow my eyes linger for few split seconds longer.

I force myself to look into her captivating eyes instead of her amazing breasts, which by the way requires incredible discipline and restraint on my part.

"I was just testing you." I tell her, with a slightly mischievous grin.

"Testing me for what?" she laughs cautiously.

"To see how you would react – I'm just doing some 'research' for my work."

"I'm glad to know you were just teasing," She says skeptically, "So what kind of work do you do? "

"I teach sign language to the blind," I tell her matter of factly while I admire the manicure on my right hand.

She pauses a second to think and says with a quizzical look, "You do what?"

"You know" I then demonstrate by faking the hand signs to the YMCA song.

"Well how can they see your hand signs if they're blind?" she laughs out loud as if I'm joking.

I look at her for a few seconds in mock disbelief. "Because I sign in cursive," I tell her…

I write cursive in the air with my finger, and I then look directly at her shaking my head. "Duh…!"

She playfully punches me in the arm.

With my devilish grin, I tell her, "But you really have to be careful when you flash signs, because one time some Mexican gang members came over wanting to know where I was from."

"Where you from ESE?" I tell her in a raspy voice using my best gangster impression. "My homeboys say they don't know where… (I quickly repeat the hand sign again) …is!"

She cracks up and looks at me as if I'm crazy. I can tell we're starting to connect. I pause and use the triangle technique again –"So enough about me - tell me about yourself – What brings you out here?" I ask her. "And don't tell me your car…"

"I don't know" – she says, "I heard this is a good place to come, meet some new people, and maybe have a few laughs…."

"Well I don't know who told you that, but you've obviously been misinformed." I firmly tell her. "This is supposed to be for adults. Didn't you see the 'No childish horseplay' sign above the door? In fact, I happen to head up the no childish horseplay committee, so keep it clean - I'd hate to have to write you up."

She laughs again - "So then what brings you out here tonight Mr. no childish horseplay?"

"I have a two seater moped" I tell her. "You probably didn't see it out front because I had it valeted, but if you're nice, I just might take you for a ride on it later." I tell her with a serious wink.

I feel an awkward moment of silence coming on, so I tell her with a slightly judgmental tone, "I don't know if I should even be hanging out with you, because you know what they say about women who wear red dresses..."

Sensing a tease, she rolls her eyes and smiles... "No, what do THEY say?"

I lean in closer as if I'm genuinely serious, and softly tell her, "They say..." I step back and look away shaking my head, "Never mind...I should have never brought it up." I chuckle.

She laughs out loud "You can't do that – What do they say?" She insists, playfully tugging on my arm.

I hesitate, weakly resist and I finally say, "OK, OK, – what they say is...," I reach for her waist and gently pull her closer to smell her hair and whisper in her ear.

"They say..." I pause again to lean back and look deeply into her eyes. "You know, you might be attractive and cool, but I don't know if I can trust you with what "They Say."

She laughs and says, "Oh, and why is that?"

I give her the Clint Eastwood squint. I look at her quizzically and tell her, "Because there's something really different about you, but I haven't yet figured it out – you're like... a mystery."

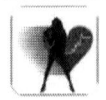

She laughs again. "A mystery? What are you talking about? No, no no no no...now you're trying to change the subject. Why do you think I'm a mystery? And don't think I'm going to forget to ask you about what 'They Say'." She says laughing. "Now you're just trying to mess with my head and confuse me..."

I move in closer again as if I'm about to share a secret. With my hand on her waist, I subtly guide and isolate her from her friends. At the same time, I move her so she is now facing only me with my back against the wall.

It now looks like she just pinned me against the wall. This maneuver causes the other women nearby to take notice, but she's not aware of it because her back is to everyone. This one subtle move now makes me seem more desirable to the rest of the women watching, as I notice more of them starting to watch me.

I tell her, "You're a mystery because you're hard to figure out... but I will. Just give me some time. In fact I'd nickname you Mister E, but since I can clearly see you're not a Mister," I approvingly look her up and down again, "I think you'd make a perfectly good Mistress E. "

Her eyes widen and she giggles, "But Mistress implies we're having an affair," she says coquettishly.

"And... So?" I wait for her response. "Remember," I admonish her, "...no childish horseplay..."

She senses I'm verbally baiting her into a trap and I can see her mind carefully searching for just the right words. "OK – I'll be mistress E if you'll be a Mister no childish horseplay," she says with a smile, "But only if you tell me what 'they say first!"

"OK, I'll tell you what Mistress E. Let's make this interesting. If you think you can correctly guess what 'They Say', or even close to it, I'll invite you over to my place to pop some grade a bubble wrap I've been saving up for just a special occasion …. That is of course IF you promise to behave yourself…"

"What?" She laughs. "Now let me get this straight…. you're going to invite me over to your place just to give me the pleasure of popping your personal stash of 'grade A' bubble wrap? –Wow – you're sweeping me off my feet," She laughs shaking her head. "But I would only come over on one condition – and that's only if I get to pop ALL of it."

"Wow – that's a pretty aggressive counter proposal…you drive a hard bargain; I'll have to think about it," I tell her with a smirk, "On the other hand, if you can't guess correctly, then…."

(To be continued…)

TABLE OF CONTENTS

INTRODUCTION: 1
  HOW TO ATTRACT WOMEN WITH HUMOR – THE DEMONSTRATION 1

CHAPTER 1 - WHY I WROTE THIS BOOK 12

CHAPTER 2 - WHAT YOU'RE GOING TO LEARN 22
  HOW TO GET THE MOST OUT OF THIS BOOK 22
  PREVIEW OF CHAPTERS 33

CHAPTER 3 - HOW I LEARNED TO ATTRACT WOMEN 37
  I KNOW THIS CAN WORK FOR YOU TOO 37
  MY EPIPHANY 42
  IT REALLY WORKS! 46
  ON THE ROAD TO FAME AND FORTUNE 47
  FURTHER PROOF THE INFORMATION WORKED 48

CHAPTER 4 - THE REASONS WOMEN ARE ATTRACTED TO MEN 51
  THE ATTRACTOR FACTORS THAT MAKE YOU DESIRABLE TO FEMALES 51
  THE SCENT OF A WOMAN 60
  HEROES AND VILLAINS 61
  LOVE THYSELF AS THY NEIGHBOR? 63
  FRIENDS AND FAMILY 64

CHAPTER 5 - HOW TO MASTER NON-VERBAL COMMUNICATION 69
  5.1 KINESICS (BODY LANGUAGE) 70
  5.2 PROXEMICS (THE USE OF SPACE) 90
  5.3 PARALANGUAGE (VOICE QUALITY OR DELIVERY) 96

CHAPTER 6 - HOW TO MASTER A SENSE OF HUMOR 100
- HERE'S HOW TO DEVELOP IT AND WHERE TO GET IT 100
- THE FACTS ABOUT PICKUP LINES 100
- THE PLAY ON WORDS 106
- OBSERVATIONAL HUMOR 109
- **UNLIMITED HUMOR ONLINE** 111
- **HUMOROUS STORY TELLING** 115
- FAKE STORY TELLING 120
- USE ANIMALS 122
- IMPRESSIONS: 124
- COLD READS 125

CHAPTER 7 - HOW TO BE THE MASTER OF APPROACHING WOMEN 128
- THE HIGH STATUS HUMOR APPROACH 132

CHAPTER 8 - HOW TO BE THE MASTER BAITER OF WOMEN 142
- HOW TO ATTRACT WOMEN AND MAKE THEM COME 142
- MALE CLEAVAGE 144
- MUTUALLY GRADUAL APPROACH 147
- MERE EXPOSURE 151
- SOCIAL EXPOSURE 152
- RESIDENTIAL PROXIMITY 154

CHAPTER 9 - THE REBIRTH OF MY LIFE AND CAREER 157
- EPILOGUE: MY BRUSH WITH DEATH AND THE LESSONS I LEARNED 157

CHAPTER 10. APPENDIX 166

ACKNOWLEDGEMENTS: 185

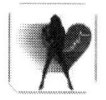

How to Attract Women With Humor

CHAPTER 1 - WHY I WROTE THIS BOOK

When I was in my early teens, I remember reading this quote from Marilyn Monroe:

"If you can get a girl to laugh, you can get her to do anything..."

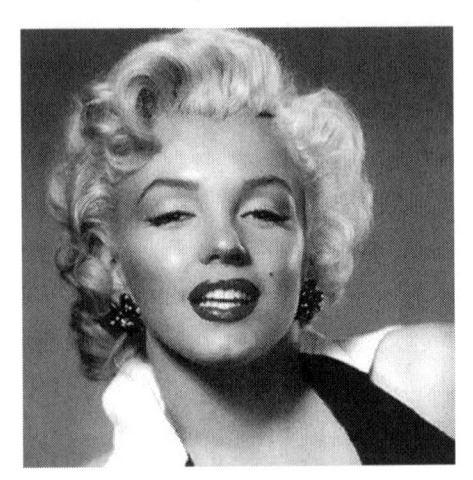

I immediately made it my mission to memorize as many jokes as I could.

In my innocent but pornographic teen mind, I imagined how I would make it work:

I'll tell her a few jokes, she'll start laughing then she'll grab me and we'll start making out. She won't be able to resist having her way with me."

I imagined in my mind, "She'll strip off her clothes and beg me to feel her up. She'll grab my hand and force me to touch her hot buttered muffin. Then, oh my god – yes –she'll beg me to insert my joystick into her game box and she'll play with it, and jiggle it, just like Sonya Blade from Mortal Kombat... until she hears the grand master say, "Finish Him!"

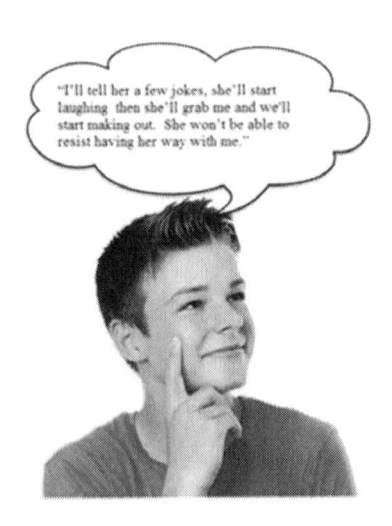

How to Attract Women With Humor

I smile to myself, "I can do this. It'll be a piece of cake."

Instead, much to my dismay – my jokes and attempts at humor resulted in a yawn and a blank stare followed by an awkward fake laugh.

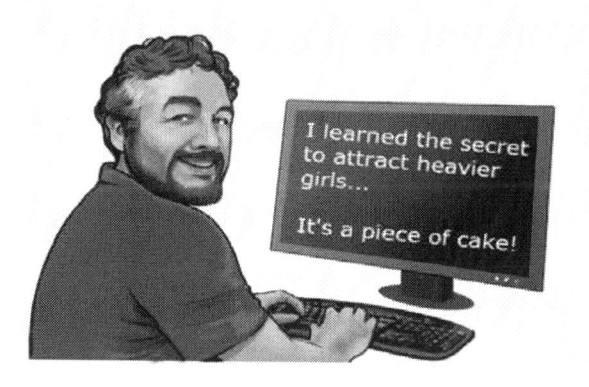

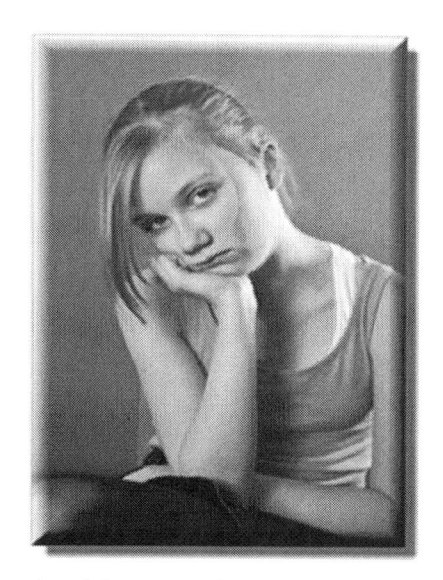

In my early teens, I was obsessed with having sex with girls. I'm sure you can relate. It was on my mind from the time I woke up with a stiff tent pole under my covers until the time I went to sleep at night.

So when I went to sleep thinking about sex, I often found my solution on hand. Unfortunately, it was from the result of and not the solution to my problem.

Maybe that's why I did so poorly in school, because all I could think of was how the girls in class would look like naked. Every last one of them – There were long ones, tall ones, short ones, brown ones, black ones, round ones, big ones, crazy ones. I even imagined all the women teachers naked, except for Ms. Schulz our history teacher who I'm sure taught WWII history from having personally experienced it.

13 | Page

How to Attract Women With Humor

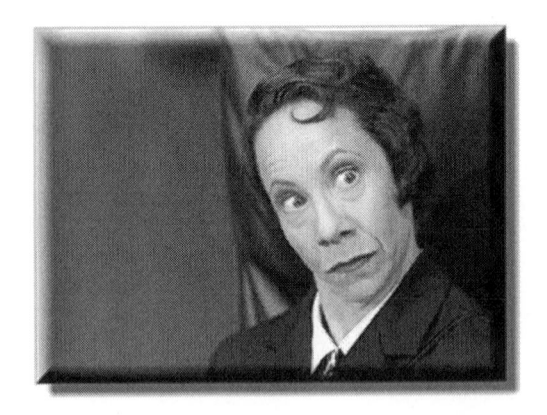

Ms. Schulz reminded me and acted a lot like , what's her name, the famous Frau Farbissina, Dr. Evil's sidekick in the Austin Powers film series. She would holler out her daily commands, "No talking and pay attention, and spit out that gum!"

What was this "lucky sensation" I felt when I imagined girls naked?

Was I the only one to feel this way? How did these feelings suddenly happen?

This all leads up to how I became such an authority on the subject. Practice, practice, practice.

When I was alone, I practiced a lot - by locking myself in the bathroom with a Sears Catalogue while I singlehandedly took on the challenge. In fact, I shook hands with the governor more times than a corrupt lobbyist on Capitol Hill.

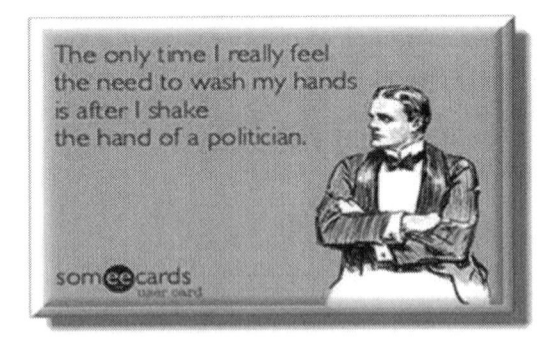

Now I could only imagine how great it would be with a real live girl. In high school and college, I played a lot of sports. I was in great shape and well liked with my teammates and male friends – but when it came to talking to girls, my mind would go blank.

14 | P a g e

This suddenly reminds me of a guy in high school who was incredibly popular with all the cutest girls - Ace Cleveland –that was his real name. Ace – Ace buddy, if you're out there – yes – I'm talking about you.

I'm sure you all knew an "Ace" in high school while growing up.

Ace was a short, little chubby guy with a bad complexion, substandard grooming habits, peach fuzzed moustache, skipped class a lot, and he wore the same trench coat nearly every day. Let's just say he wasn't the brightest crayon in the box.

It was clear he was not destined to be the academic standard-bearer for institutions of higher education. If he was ever fortunate enough to even land a job, it would probably be one with his nametag stitched above his shirt pocket. No offense if this describes you; even I had one of those jobs growing up. If you're already grown and you still have it, then let's just move on.

Nevertheless, the girls always wanted to be with him! He seemed to have different girlfriend every month, and when they went out on dates, they would pay!

What did he have that I didn't? Why did all the cute girls like him more than me? I was much cuter (at least in my mind I was) and I could easily kick his ass. I studied him in action with girls, but at the time, I couldn't figure out how he did it. In retrospect and after much research, I finally broke the code.

I realize now the reason that cute girls wanted to be with him so much was his natural ability to playfully tease and challenge them in a humorous way.

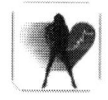

Meanwhile, it seemed the nicer and friendlier I tried to be with girls; the more they tried to avoid me or want to be "just friends." Even though I had a lot more going for me at the time, (like a Honda 50 motorcycle and a job making pizzas) this made me realize that with young girls, personality trumps appearance and status nearly every time.

As a senior in high school, I finally landed a hot girl friend, Kathy Lewis; and the first time we made love, I knew I had found my purpose in life. It was the most incredible 2.7 seconds I ever experienced. I was so in love. I put her on a pedestal and I did everything she wanted.

After a few months, I noticed she began losing interest in me. She soon became more interested in my best friend, and you can probably guess what happened next, the triple whammy. She came to me one day and said, "We need to take a break. It's not you, it's me, but I still like you as a friend."

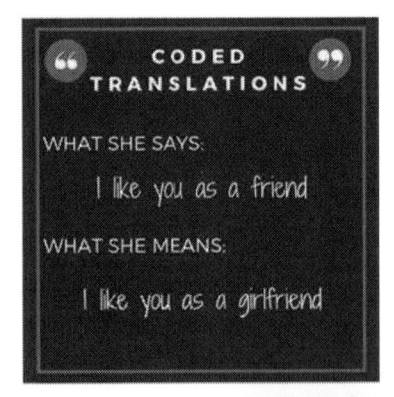

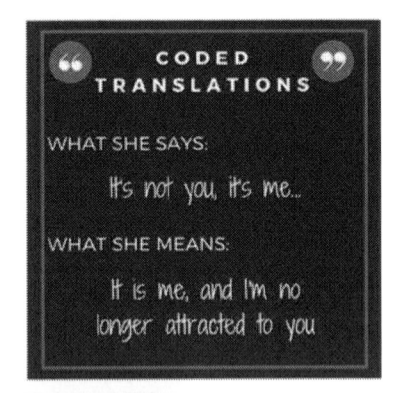

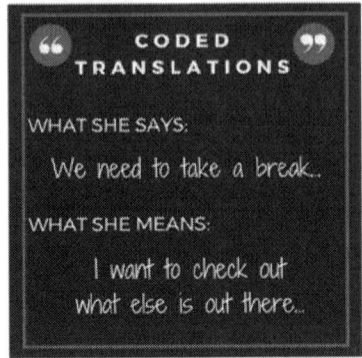

CODED TRANSLATIONS

WHAT SHE SAYS:
I like you as a friend

WHAT SHE MEANS:
I like you as a girlfriend

CODED TRANSLATIONS

WHAT SHE SAYS:
It's not you, it's me...

WHAT SHE MEANS:
It is me, and I'm no longer attracted to you

CODED TRANSLATIONS

WHAT SHE SAYS:
We need to take a break...

WHAT SHE MEANS:
I want to check out what else is out there...

Now here are the coded translations if you want to know. Here's what she says, "I like you as a friend." Here's what she means, "I like you as a girlfriend." What she says, "It's not you, it's me." What she means, "It is me, and I'm no longer attracted to you."

Coded Translation 3 - What she says: "We need to take a break." What she means, "I want to check out what else is out there…"

I was devastated, crushed, and humiliated – it was the worst feeling I ever experienced in my life. I was sick for months.

If you have ever had your heart broken, then you know how it feels. Within a few months of being with Kathy, I went from the highest high to the absolute lowest low.

I never wanted to feel that way again. This created in me the desire to learn everything I could about attracting the best women possible and make them want me so much that they would never want to leave me. It would be perfectly ok if I left them however.

I eventually found the answers through many years of research and experimentation. I discovered that much of attraction has to do with evolutionary psychology and learning how and why men and women draw each other at a primal level. Women want men who will make them feel good, feel protected, add value to their lives, and have the resources and/or status to make them want to stay.

Throughout this book, I'll be sharing with you some outrageous stories that will help you to attract women and make them feel good, along with some tragically pitiful ones that will help you to avoid the mistakes I've made. These are lessons I learned that I'm sure some of you have already experienced, or to at least you can relate.

I can tell you that after several years of mistakes, heartaches, research, and practice, I eventually learned how to attract and be with a number of incredibly gorgeous and sexy women. Lots of them – and I became good enough to appear on TV, radio, get featured in national publications and even give advice to a very large audience on a nationally syndicated radio program.

I discovered that it takes more than just memorizing a few jokes. You need to learn how to cultivate attractive humor so you can approach women with the proper eye contact, body language, confidence, and delivery if you want to make them attracted to you.

All it takes is the ability to make some minor adjustments in your body language, mindset, and have the willingness to practice some of the techniques and information you'll learn here so you can adapt it to your own style and personality.

High Status Humor or attractive humor is the best type of icebreaker to spark attraction with women because it instantly short-circuits their internal defense mechanism. She will quickly come to trust and like you more when you naturally tap into the emotional part of her brain.

It's important to know that there is a major difference between "Low Status" and "High Status Humor." Low status humor is acting like Carrot Top, Gallagher, or Don Rickles. Although it might get women to laugh at you, it probably won't get you laid a lot.

Now think of the type of humor 007 James Bond, Charlie Harper from Two and a Half Men, or Chandler Bing from Friends might use. That's High Status Humor. It's the difference between them laughing with you and not at you.

Learning playful and challenging banter – also known as flirting - has allowed me to have several incredible romantic and sexual experiences – the kind that flash before you on your deathbed.

Coincidentally, I also learned that you can experience even more pleasure with beautiful women than just sex itself (of course that is a major component); like getting to know, trust and intimately connect with a woman on a deep, emotional level. I know that this disclosure may come as a surprise to some of you, but it truly takes sexual pleasure to the ultimate level.

I want this book to be more than just a guide on how to pick up women just so you can move on to the next one. You're shortchanging yourself if you think that's the objective. Sure, it might be fun for a while, but you'll eventually discover the ultimate pleasure comes from having a deeply intimate sexual relationship.

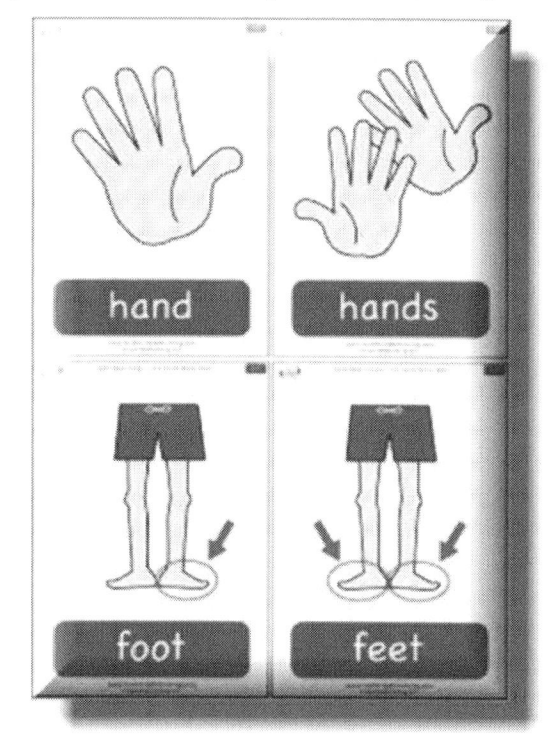

I want to help you not only attract women to make them want you, but also to give you the tools to connect on a deeper level; because just like the hokey pokey, that's what it's all about.

You want to live, laugh, and love her at the deepest and most vulnerable levels especially during passionate lovemaking because eventually once you experience the difference you'll begin to discover that having just a one night stand is not enough room to put all your devices on when you go to sleep.

High Status Humor has also helped me to succeed in business and my social life because it can be a very powerful tool to influence others to make them like and trust you. It's also very useful to sell others your ideas too.

If you have ever kicked yourself for not approaching an attractive woman you wanted to meet because you chickened out or didn't know how, or if you've ever had a great rapport going with a woman and then she suddenly lost interest in you; then use this information so you won't have to experience those types of situations ever again.

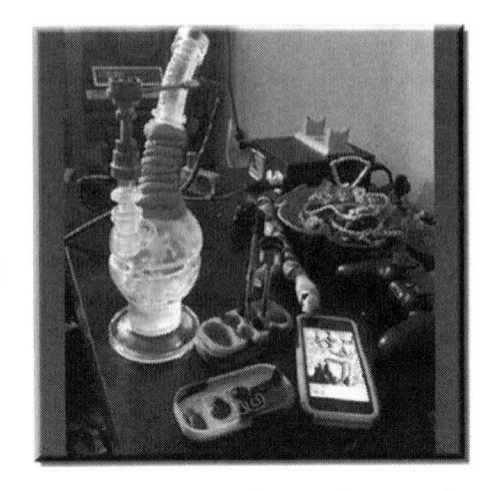

Based on decades of experiments, scientific research, the experiences of other experts as well as my own; this information is truly the art and science of attracting high quality women so you can create a fun and exciting connection with them. When you master these techniques, you'll never have these problems again.

By the time you finish this book, you'll be able to easily approach practically any woman, practically anytime, practically anywhere with supreme confidence, and establish a very powerful and humorous connection with her.

If you want to have awesome relationships with the highest quality women, then you must first learn the psychology and fundamentals of approaching them in a way that sparks instant attraction. You only get one chance to make a good first impression, and there's a high probability you may not get a second one. Why take months and years when you can get the ball rolling right away?

You'll never even get to first base unless you learn how to step up to the plate and properly prepare for the pitch. Only then can you regularly hit home runs and the occasional "Grand Slam" where you can score four with one pitch, a pitch that I'll demonstrate in the upcoming pages.

Playing the field and one-night stands can be fun for a while, but eventually, I truly believe you'll want to settle down with one, at least for a few years. Once you find her, there is nothing better than to share true love and sex in its highest and purest form the type that you can only experience from a longer-term relationship.

This book promises to show you how to increase your confidence and use high status attractive humor, body language and eye contact to make women want to be with you so you too can have countless memorable and unforgettable encounters with lots of beautiful, sexy women throughout your life.

When you get good enough, you'll discover that women will then start approaching you!

I hope you will enjoy reading this as much as I enjoyed writing it and reliving some of my adventures with the various wonderful sexy and beautiful women throughout my life.

CHAPTER 2 - WHAT YOU'RE GOING TO LEARN

HOW TO GET THE MOST OUT OF THIS BOOK

Throughout this course, I've posted several cartoons with humorous lines that you can begin to use right away to start conversations. I've also included other images and techniques to help you keep conversations interesting and humorous.

I'll be sharing personal anecdotes as examples to help you incorporate the advice and content in a natural way so you can blend it with your own style and personality.

I want you to start employing right away some simple, masculine, non-verbal communication skills I'm going to teach so you can immediately gain more confidence. Your whole life changes once you begin to notice when women start paying more attention to you.

One of the keys to attracting women when you first meet them is learning how to project your body language while deciphering theirs. For women that you already know and associate with, it will be even that much easier to engage them in fun and humorous storytelling because there is familiarity already built in. High status humor or affiliative humor breeds familiarity.

The more you do it, the easier it will become and the more your confidence will soar because of your success. As women start paying you more attention, more opportunities will present themselves. One will continue to enhance the other until it becomes natural.

It will first take some practice and the willingness to step a little out of your comfort zone to master, but it definitely will be worth it in the end. It will change your life.

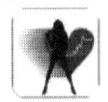

For the beginners who have not yet developed the confidence, I'm going to share with you a simple approach to meet attractive women that I first used when I started. I have used it successfully over a hundred times since and **it never failed even once** to engage women in a fun and exciting, humorous conversation; and it's so easy!

This straightforward approach allows you to engage instantly in a fun and fascinating conversation based on the questions that become part of it. It is so dynamic that right after I finish this book, my next one will be on the use and implementation of this incredible technique.

Sign up for my free dating tips at the end or at the beginning and I'll give you a sneak peak.

It's no secret that the most successful guys who easily attract women use cocky and funny dialogue to start conversations. Marilyn Monroe was right when she made her comment about making women laugh; however, she should have added the disclaimer that it also must also include using high status humor with congruent body language if you want to yield optimum results.

She failed to mention that by the way.It would have saved me lots of embarrassment.

I'm going to break down the approach step by step and analyze it so you can see exactly how it's done and why it is so effective. The intro demonstration was an actual case scenario and I'm going to use it as the example to give you a behind the scenes peek.

t the end of this book, you will find in the appendix several humorous openers and follow-up passages you can use to develop high status humor so you can become the man that women want. Once you combine alpha male habits to establish her welcoming eye contact and body language, the rest is effortless and lots of fun.

Remember, the vast majority of men who are successful with women use playful, cocky, and funny humor.

For example, here is an easy opener that I have used, it's my hip pocket approach:

Nice red shoes, I have a pair just like them...

then follow up with a cold read,

You know what they say about girls who wear red shoes...

or you could follow with a humorous question,

Didn't I see your dating profile on redshoes.com or was it Farmer's only.com? Which one was it, because I was on both...?

Once you break the ice with a humorous opener coupled with confident body language and eye contact, you short-circuit her brain to bypass the awkward stage that most guys fail to get past. You immediately become more likeable when you make her laugh, even if it's a stupid joke.

You can easily learn a few humorous responses to typical questions you know they will ask you...,

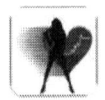

Q: How are you?

A: I had a long accident at the mall today; I fell down an up escalator...

She may ask you,

Q: What do you do?

Tell her,

A: I own a chain of discount self-service massage parlors...

You can have her instantly laughing at your own humorous personal experiences when you know how to set them up properly. These are the same ones you've already told your family and friends lots of times, you just have to know how to set them up in these encounters..

Or, you could talk about dating and take a conversation into a totally different direction...

I stopped dating this one girl because she used too many 4-letter words, like – Stop! Don't! and Quit That! She wanted me to treat her like royalty so I took her to Burger King and Diary Queen...

I've even posted several quips you can use to escalate an encounter so you can playfully "take it to the next level," but of course, you should only use these after you've established a connection.

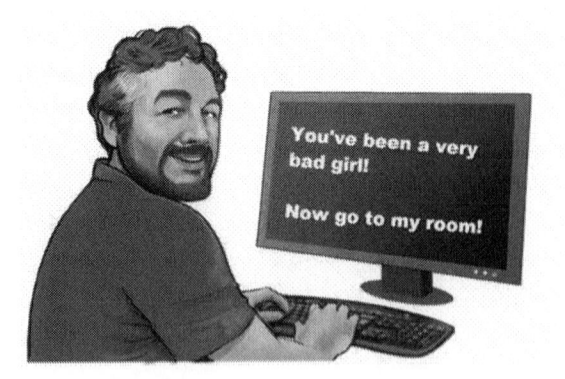

These are only a few of many openers and follow-ups you can use, but just using them is only a small part of the process. I will also provide you with a number of entertaining ways to keep conversations amusing, fun, and interesting.

I will take you through a step-by-step process to show you the proper mindset, setup, body language, eye contact; content and delivery you'll need to know so that you can approach and make women want to be with you.

Once you practice and master these techniques, it's like walking or riding a bicycle. It will become effortless and you won't even have to think about it. It will become routine, like learning to drive a stick shift; which then becomes automatic.

In order to become the type of man that women are naturally attracted to, it's so much easier when you have a role model like George Clooney, Vince Vaughan, or Charlie Sheen you can emulate to adapt to your own style.

By purchasing this book, I hereby give you permission to use even me as your role model but only IF you purchase my course first. I have to warn you that I have trained a squadron of infiltrators to be on the lookout for imposters who have not yet purchased the full course and are unauthorized to impersonate me or use my material.

As you may have noticed, I don't joke around. You can find more information about my courses by signing up for my free dating tips at the end.

Now I'm definitely not suggesting that you need to become the same person as the role model or become anyone other than yourself. I am suggesting that after learning this process, you should incorporate the mannerisms and style of the person you'd most like to model yourself after – and use their persona to develop your own personal style of machismo.

Anyone who has ever accomplished anything of significance in life modeled himself or herself after someone and oftentimes many others they admired. That's all I'm asking you to do.

Modeling yourself after someone whom you think is your perfect role model you'd like to emulate can help you to become the best version of

yourself much faster. It also makes the process much easier.

My buddy William Shakespeare once said, "All the world's a stage, and all the men and women merely players; they have their exits and their entrances, and one man in his time plays many parts."

Let's examine this concept for a moment, especially those of you who may be skeptical of this approach and may not be open to trying something new.

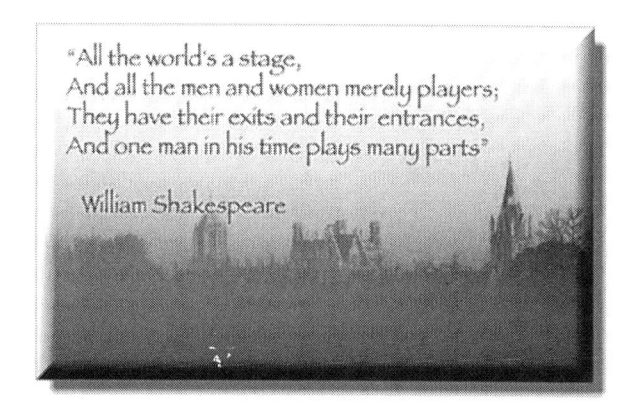

"All the world's a stage,
And all the men and women merely players;
They have their exits and their entrances,
And one man in his time plays many parts"

William Shakespeare

Do you act and speak to young children the same way you do adults? Do you talk to a panhandler the same way you do your boss? Would you address an annoying neighbor you're trying to avoid the same way you would a new girl you're trying to impress, or a telemarketer you're trying to get rid of versus a cop you're trying to talk out of a traffic ticket?

You have learned through your life's experiences how to relate to others depending on the situation and your desired outcome.

The point I'm trying to make is we all adapt our personalities, our body language, what and how we say things that depend on the type of person we're talking to and what we're trying to accomplish.

I'm certainly not suggesting that you need to memorize a script like lines in a play, but I do suggest that you can learn to play off all the props that surround you and create humor from the rich history of your own life experiences and the funny circumstances that happen every day of your life.

Alternatively, you have permission to use any of the lines I've posted in the appendix to start out with until you begin to accumulate a repertoire of your own. The key is to start becoming aware of opportunities to create humor in things that you experience every day.

Your life will be easier and much more rewarding when you begin to learn how to find humor in places where you least expect it, like moments of anger, pain and conflict. In the long run, you will feel better, live longer, make more friends, and certainly meet a lot more women.

When you're about to give a presentation or speak to a new client or group of people – do you just wing it– or do you have something prepared like a planned conversation or outline that you've mentally rehearsed and practiced beforehand?

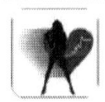

Which process do you think will give you a higher level of confidence and results that are more successful? Why not become the most desirable, attractive and humorous version of yourself by using every tool at your disposal so you can win more women and influence people?

The more you practice your presentation, the more successful you will become. This includes the mastery of your body language, eye contact, content, and delivery; and it's a lot easier to do than you might think.

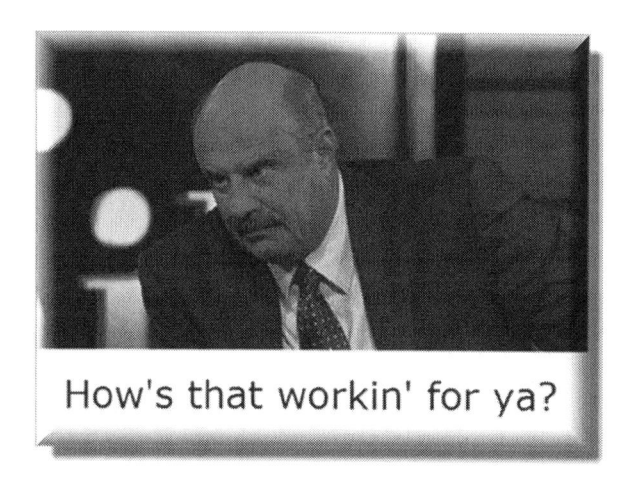

Just think of what you have to gain! If you haven't had much success with what you're currently doing, I'd like to quote Dr. Phil:

How's that workin' for ya?

Master these techniques and your life will drastically improve not only with women, but also with practically everyone you meet. Others will like and trust you more quickly when you're able to put them at ease and make them laugh naturally with high status humor.

I'm happy for the women's liberation movement and equality, but with it became the feminization of American society. The Equal Rights Movement for women in the 60's has caused role reversals and gender confusion that contradicts the conditioning of tens of thousands of years of customary male-female roles.

Male and female blueprints that took around 200,000 years to evolve upended suddenly over the last 50. That is a 4,000 to 1 ratio! That's like starting on less than the 1-inch line on a football field of a hundred yards. It's no wonder the modern male population is so confused.

In many ways, traditional male and female roles are no longer relevant and the sudden shift has had major social consequences. One of the primary reasons so many feminized males (often referred to as wusses) are unsuccessful in attracting women is they act like women themselves.

It does not work. You can't reverse a few hundred thousand years of conditioning over a 50-year period and expect different results.

At the same time, it's been proven in studies that many women who *think and say* they desire sensitive, emotional, nice guys – (who are in reality, feminized men), are actually attracted to masculine men who are not sensitive or emotional at all.

Research showed that when those women met men in speed dating encounters, overwhelmingly they chose the men who displayed the alpha male traits and turned down the passive sensitive men.

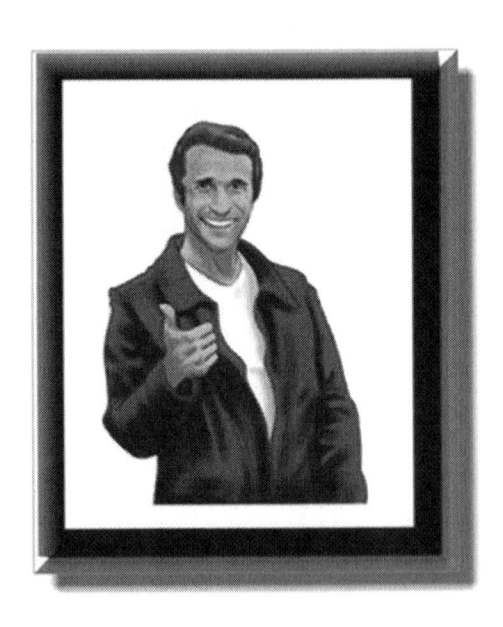

On the one hand, it wouldn't be prudent to grab women by their hair and drag them back to your man cave as we previously noted. It would be "uncivilized" and you would find yourself on Fox News debating Gloria Allred.

On the other hand, you have four fingers and a thumb

Heeeyyyy

just like the Fonz to reclaim your masculinity so you can display the Attractor Factors that will cause women to become subconsciously attracted to you.

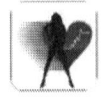

There was a time when attractive females intimidated me. I tended to put women on a pedestal, bought them lots of gifts, took them to great restaurants and treated them like princesses.

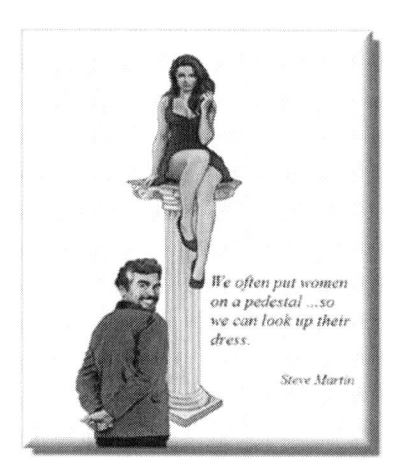

The amount of time and money I spent trying to score was staggering. Even though I had much going for me at the time, I still struck out more times than Babe Ruth (who by the way also held the record for the most home runs for a long time).

I started practicing and using more Masculine Body Language. I started improving everything I could about myself. I started developing more self-respect and confidence. I also stopped trying so hard to please women and that made a huge difference. However, the real catalyst to this magic formula was developing and integrating a confident sense of high status humor.

As I became more successful, I immediately noticed that the people I met were friendlier and started treating me with more respect, including my family and friends.

Women I encountered started smiling more and making longer eye contact. I began to engage nearly everyone I met to hone my humor skills, and it became a lot of fun.

More people started calling me "sir," because of the way others

respectfully treated me. The more I practiced these newfound habits, the more self-confidence I began to develop. I started memorizing and modifying a repertoire of funny bits used by famous comedians that gave me more confidence to start developing my own style of humor to make women laugh.

I'm going to teach you how to start developing your own style of humor, and when used with alpha male body language and habits, you'll be amazed at the way others will start treating you. You will

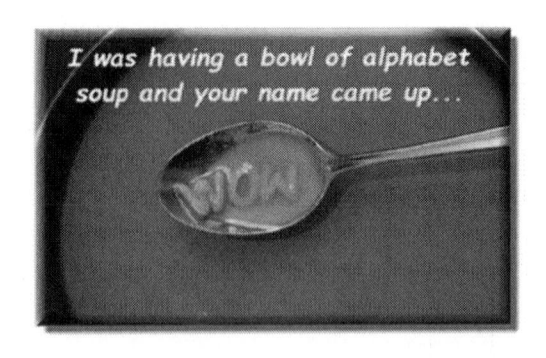

> *I was having a bowl of alphabet soup and your name came up...*

genuinely look forward to interacting with more people because it's fun and entertaining to make folks laugh.

With a little practice, you will start noticing that women will start to smile more at you because of the way they feel when you make them laugh. You'll especially notice how they will start engaging you in a more playful manner. You'll find that women will begin to introduce you to their girlfriends and they will all want to start spending more time with you.

The purpose of this book is to show you how to develop the traits that cause others (especially women) to notice and respect you more. You grew up with a modern "female blueprint" and I'm going to show you how to record over it. In fact, starting today, I want you to relearn and start demonstrating right away the modern masculine characteristics women can't help but become attracted.

The methods you're about to learn were scientifically tested and proven to work in social experiments. This information has been carefully researched and documented from experts in the fields of evolutionary psychology, sociology, neuroscience, evolutionary biology, anthropology, and many other fields too numerous to mention.

First, I want to make one thing clear. I don't pretend to have the magic formula that works for every man with every woman. No single prescription fits every situation. Countless methods truly work in various types of situations. What I've done is to focus on the common denominators and fundamentals that are effective with the widest array of women and at their deepest emotional level of wants and needs.

Your goal is to make women like, trust and respect you; and that type of connection comes when you can create a humorous and positive atmosphere that they will come to have fun in and enjoy.

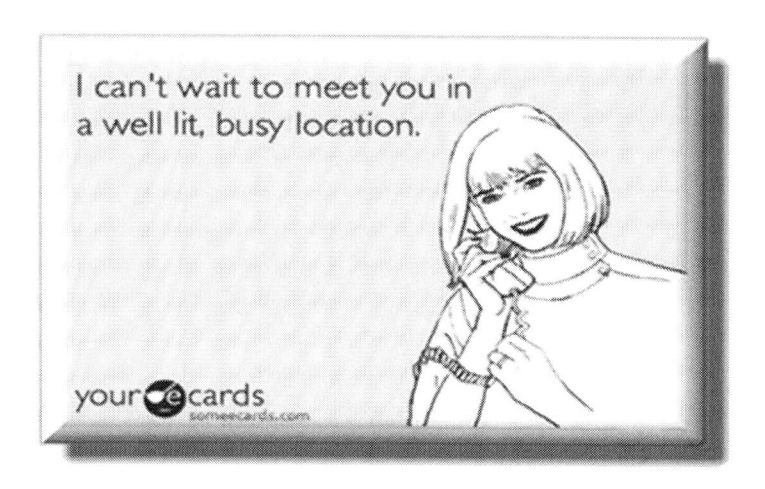

> I can't wait to meet you in a well lit, busy location.
>
> your ecards
> someecards.com

PREVIEW OF CHAPTERS

Every day of your life can provide limitless opportunities to make a lasting impact on women you wish to impress for romantic, business, or social purposes. Many men realize all of the positive qualities and attributes they have; sometimes some may have trouble bringing them out.

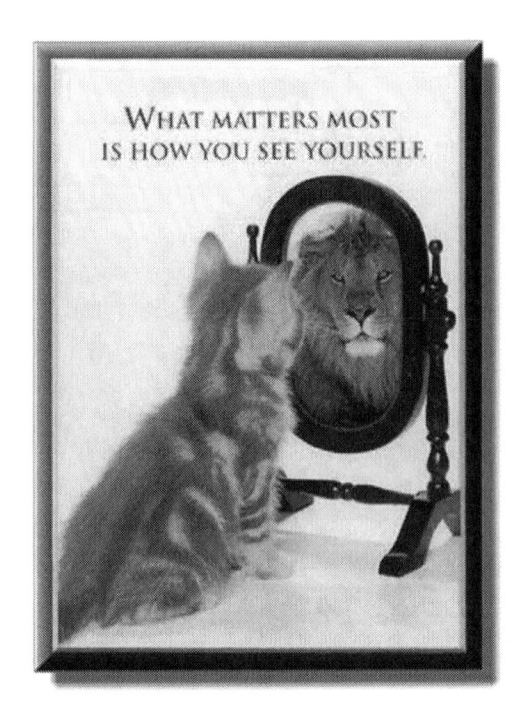

You need to reclaim your natural masculinity! One of my favorite things in life is to engage an attractive woman in a playful, flirtatious conversation and experience the incredible sensation that overcomes you when you connect in a way that creates desire between you.

In the first chapter *"How I learned to attract women"* I'm going to tell you my story and the steps I took to learn how to attract women. I'm going to reveal the patented line I created that enabled me to approach ANY woman I wanted to meet easily, with total confidence and without fear.

This simple method will blow you away when you realize how easy and foolproof it is. I'm proud to be its creator, and I hereby certify I've never seen it used before by anyone else in any of the research I've conducted over 30 plus years.

In the second chapter, *"The Reasons Women are Attracted to Men,"* reveals the evolutionary history and explains why sex has been the major factor of humans becoming the dominant species on earth, and how men developed certain traits, or "attractor factors" throughout history to attract women.

You'll learn what those "ornaments" are and why women are attracted to them at the subconscious and primal level. Just as you are attracted to a beautiful face, ass and breasts, so are women attracted to "male cleavage", or attractor factors that I'm going to show you how to develop. Men's cues for sex are visual while women's cues are psychological.

In the third chapter, *"How to Master Non Verbal Communication"* I'm going to show you how to develop the body language, eye contact and touching cues that women cannot help but become irresistibly attracted to. You don't need to be rich or good lucking to make them work either.

In the fourth chapter, *"How to be the Master of Humor"* I show you several ways how you can easily develop an awesome sense of high status humor that fits your own personality so you can use it to not only attract more women, but to get others to like and trust you more.

In the fifth chapter, *"How to be the Master Baiter of Women,"* I'm going to show you how to make women come, so you don't have to do all the work. I'm going to reveal the 12 habits of the Human Alpha Male – the attractor factors that been scientifically proven to attract women to you instead of you having to always approach them first.

By the time you finish this book you will have discovered some amazing revelations about female evolutionary psychology and human behavior. You will learn the subconscious and hidden secret desires of women so you can make use of them to become irresistible. This information will cause you to better understand and totally rethink the way you relate and talk to them.

You'll discover how high status humor can become an aphrodisiac for women when it puts them into an instant and emotional state of attraction when done properly. You'll learn how to keep a conversation interesting and how to transition into thoughtful personal dialogue that builds deep rapport.

So let's begin with my story…

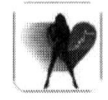

CHAPTER 3 - HOW I LEARNED TO ATTRACT WOMEN

I KNOW THIS CAN WORK FOR YOU TOO

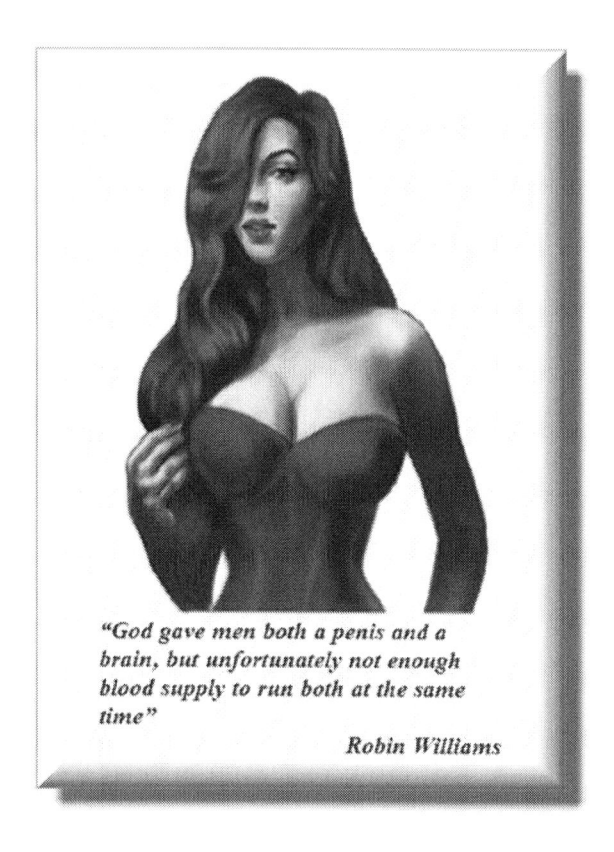

"God gave men both a penis and a brain, but unfortunately not enough blood supply to run both at the same time"

Robin Williams

Robin Wlliams once said, "God gave men both a penis and a brain, but unfortunately not enough blood supply to run both at the same time.

In 1978, Playboy Magazine ranked San Diego State University one of the top three partying schools in the country, which I can personally verify because I lived it.

I was a graduate student at the time, and all I could focus on were the stunningly gorgeous girls with tanned firm bodies parading around campus. I vividly recall the seductive way their hips swayed and the vision of their breathtakingly beautiful apricot asses that peeked out the bottom of their high cut tight shorts.

These cuddly co-eds typically wore see through form fitting halter-tops with no bras and they made sure to bounce when they walked. Their firm breasts jiggled like jello begging to be motor boated. They loved to tease and give flirtatious come-hither glances.

I felt so helpless - talk about focus stealers. When I gawked at them, I was unable to study or carry on a conversation without words freezing in mid sentence or my mind turning blank. I was then compelled to find the nearest restroom and find an empty stall so I could shake hands with my best friend.

The urge to reach out and touch these tempting vixens was overwhelming. It was all I could think of. I wanted to get close to them, to know them, to touch them, to kiss them and get naked.

The urge was so strong, and even with my college level research skills I was unable to find any literature to teach me how to coax these women into my bedroom.

Sure there were sporadic articles in Playboy, Penthouse and even Cosmo that had a few tips on how to meet girls, but there was really only one book I could find on the subject at the time "How to Pick up Girls" by Eric Weber and you could only buy it through a display ad he placed in Playboy Magazine.

It was a huge seller at the time. He became famous and he was all over the radio and TV. So I ordered a copy and I couldn't wait to read it. The "book" was about 68 pages long, the width of about 3 and a half quarters. It had large print with lots of pictures.

Since he was the first person I found to write such a book, I really have to give him credit for creating this revolutionary, niche market manuscript, even though the content pales in comparison to the volumes of today that contain much more effective information on attracting women.

Since I was working on my Master's degree at the time, I talked to one of my college professors about my interest in this subject and I informed him of the lack of any real good or specific information on how to attract women.

I was positive I could write a better book than Weber's on picking up girls. The bachelor professor confirmed that it was subject matter worthy of a class project. However if it was to be considered a valid research project commendable of receiving course credit, it would need to be scientific in nature and provide sources with footnotes.

Part of my research was to conduct surveys and ask many questions. What better source of answers could I find on attracting women than asking opinions of attractive women?

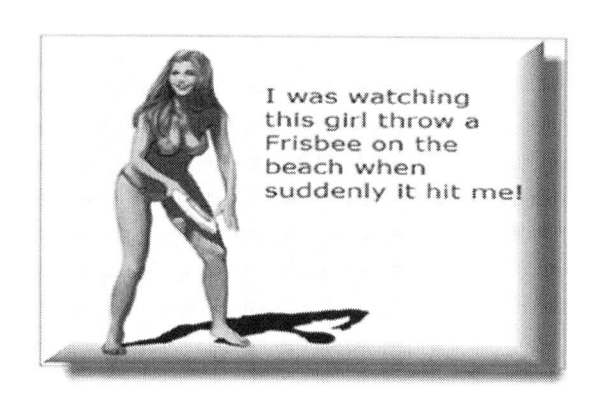

I was watching this girl throw a Frisbee on the beach when suddenly it hit me!

I could use my research as a justification to meet women! I carefully constructed the following question that would allow me to approach any woman fearlessly. Whenever I saw an attractive woman I wanted to meet, I would approach her and ask the following question, which henceforth I will officially dub "Leonardo's Lead-in." I would approach her sincerely and say:

> *"I picked you out of everyone because you seem like the perfect female to ask...I'm writing a book on love and attraction. Do you have a few moments, and would you be so kind as to give me your opinion on a few quick simple questions I have?"*

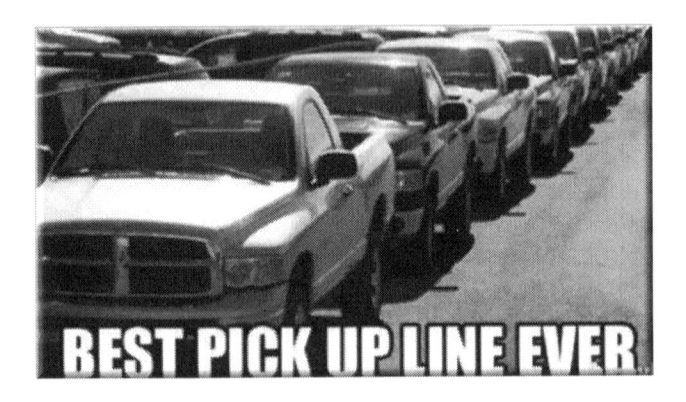

BEST PICK UP LINE EVER.

What "perfect" woman doesn't like to talk about love and attraction? What woman isn't going take just a few moments to "give you her opinion" and answer a few, quick, simple questions? I would then began to ask flirtatious, penetrating questions disguised as research that led to humor, attraction, a phone number, a date, a massage, etc...

You can slightly modify this lead-in to make it work for you. For example, you could change, "I'm writing a book on" to

- "I'm doing research on" or
- "I have a bet with a friend" or
- "I'm in a contest to get the best answers" or
- "I'm conducting a survey" or even
- "I have an assignment on."

Because you are reading this book, I hereby give you this assignment; so now you're not lying. Now, don't you think you can ask that non-threatening question to approach literally *any* woman you want to meet who has a few minutes? It's so easy!

In my upcoming course "Leonardo's Lead-in," I'm going to give you the complete program on how to use this foolproof technique. I'm going to include all of the follow-up questions you can ask that are psychologically designed to engage her in a fun, interesting, deep and meaningful conversation which you can use to intimately get to know her the first time you meet.

You won't believe how easy and natural it is to "escalate" the relationship once you get her to disclose intimate details of her life. It's been proven that disclosing deeply personal details of one's life can't help but make one closer to the person being disclosed to. Psychologists call this observable fact transference.

The proper touching during these times serves to magnify the experience, and makes it easier for the person to disclose. It's been proven that we are much more likely to open up to a person more when there is touching involved, but there has to be a reason for touching. For example, women are more likely to gab about their personal life to a hair stylist, manicurist, or masseuse.

The same goes for men. It's so much easier to talk to somebody who is touching you, but for a reason. Once I begin to use this lead-in, I now had the confidence, the perfect opener and I was unstoppable. It was Showtime! I modestly admit that I became a very smooth, sexcessful, fearless love machine.

Of course, women welcomed the approach because it was simple, it didn't seem like a pickup at all. It felt natural, and I never met a woman who didn't have an interest in love and attraction. If they were "good," I promised, I "might" even mention them in the book.

It was the best pickup line ever! Not even one time did it ever fail to generate attraction or interest from any women I approached, ever.

I soon developed a repertoire of flirtatious follow up questions and storytelling of my own that made meeting a girl for the first time effortless and that led to many memorable encounters. In fact, I randomly approached women just to try out new material for the fun of it even if I did not intend to ask for a phone number or a date.

MY EPIPHANY

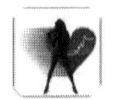

There's that old saying that all good things must end. My adventurous "research" methods culminated one fateful warm summer evening in my macho bachelor pad near the beach in Ventura.

Talk about the perfect storm.

I was entertaining a young hottie in my bedroom who I just met at the beach. Suddenly the front door bell and the phone in my bedroom rang almost simultaneously. I was irritated over the coitus interruptus, but that was nothing compared to what was about to happen next.

The abrupt sound of glass shattering followed by the shrill sound of a car alarm-wailing outside my bedroom window unexpectedly interrupted my blissful day. I couldn't decide to run first to the phone, the front door, or the bedroom window.

I chose the window, jumped out of bed naked, and ran to see just in time one of the girls I was "dating" burning rubber screeching off furiously in her car out of the parking lot.

I yelled "What the hell? She just put a brick through my windshield!" I was then horror-struck to discover that I left my bedroom blinds cracked open just enough to see a clear path from the window to my bed.

Damshitfuck.

My new ex girlfriend in the bed couldn't help but notice my eyes swivel back and forth a few times from the open blinds to the bed. I'm sure she could figure it out, I was busted. She pulled back the covers and began to look nervously around the room for her clothes.

As she was getting dressed, we both could not help but overhear the voices over my answering machine. "This is Leonardo; leave a message at the beep!"

"Leo, this is Cindi - care to come over tonight and play doctor? I need an examination... Call me!"

Cindi led two lives – Cindi the conservative, Republican church going good girl, and the one I came to know intimately between the sheets. Fearful of her reputation, she used to tell her friends and family we were just "dating."

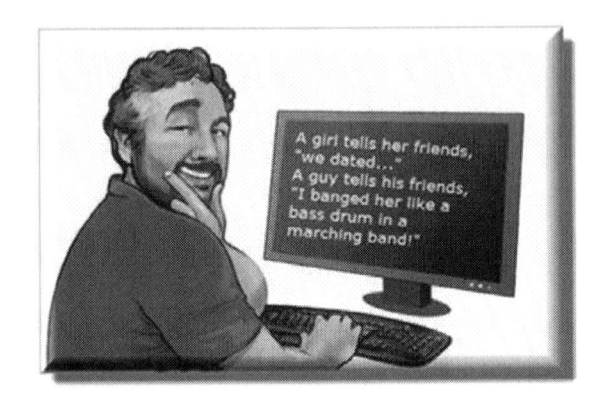

As Cindi finished hanging up, I heard the voice of my next-door neighbor Misty, a slightly older eccentric busty blonde bombshell who was still in her prime. She was outside my front door ringing the doorbell. "Yoo Hoo – Leonardo – are you home?"

I'm assuming this was too much drama for the young lady I was entertaining in my bedroom (sorry, I forgot her name) because she hurriedly dressed and bolted for the front door without even stopping to say goodbye...or even a well-deserved hug or thank you... or at least a peck on the cheek.

As the young hottie frantically exited stage right out my front door, she left the door open enough for my eccentric neighbor Misty to come in, and as if on cue, she made her dramatic entrance inside.

My head was spinning around like Regan's in the scene from the Exorcist.

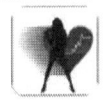

Just like in a Broadway play, she gracefully glides into the room and elevates her hand to the sky, then elegantly brings her elbows to rest on my counter top. She props her face in her palms with a big smile and says, "So whatcha doin'?"

She was dressed in a very sheer unbuttoned robe, and she gave me "the look." Since I became accustomed to giving her a "neighborly welcome" since the first time she "borrowed a cup of sugar," she began to come over more frequently unannounced. This time she came dressed only in a sexy nightgown revealing more than her intentions.

For a split second, my mind impulsively thought of maneuvering her into the bedroom. Fortunately, (or unfortunately depending on which head is in control) the head that can type and tell a story prevailed. I came to my senses and decided instead to try to repair the damage and crisis unfolding around me.

I'm just glad my long distance girlfriend didn't happen to pop in unannounced that day. That would have been catastrophic. She was as gorgeous as she was unforgiving. You probably would not be reading this book had fate intervened that day with her finding out because I would not have been alive to write it.

I think God was trying to send me a warning.

That night I had one of those life-changing epiphanies when I paused to look at myself naked in the mirror. I had not been getting much sleep or eating right. I was drinking way too much. My face was pale, puffy and I had a 3-day stubble.

There were big bags under my bloodshot eyes – bags big enough to pack and leave town for a few days, a thought that temporarily crossed my mind. I looked down at my pride and joy –the one-eyed monster. I firmly grasped him and looked him right in the eye. Weak from attrition, he dangled helplessly like an MMA fighter too late to tap out from a rear naked chokehold.

"Arrgh I growled - What's wrong with you?" as I shook him. "This is another fine mess you've gotten me into!" I had to figure out how to extricate myself tactfully from another conundrum that I now found myself.

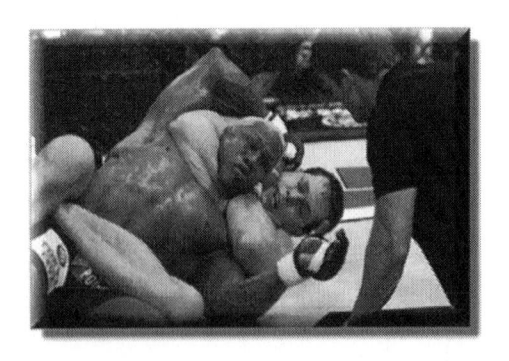

I had become a man whore. Yes – I was "dating" four women at once, the proverbial grand slam. Oddly enough, the more I began to ponder my dilemma and think back on my teen years, the more my shame started to subside.

In fact, to be honest I started to become rather amused and proud of my accomplishments. I began to smile sheepishly as I started to recount the many encounters. I took out a piece of paper and started writing them down. I may have even blushed a time or two while shaking my head.

One thing for sure, you could say it taught me a lesson - everything in moderation...But this was my momentous epiphany:

IT REALLY WORKS!

At that moment, I felt like I just discovered the cure for cancer! I will become rich and famous - a savior to all mankind. I pictured Wayne and Garth kneeling and bowing in front of me.

How to Attract Women With Humor

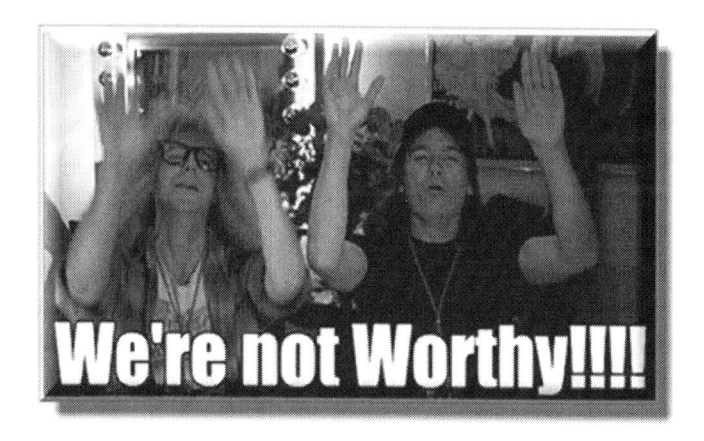

"We're not worthy, we're not worthy!"

Delusions of grandeur flooded my brain because I just knew I was on to something new – a formula that men would pay a fortune to learn.

ON THE ROAD TO FAME AND FORTUNE

I eventually became more judicious with my behavior when I finally published the book. I promoted it through speaking engagements and book signings. Personalities interviewed me on television and radio shows – Journalists featured me in newspapers and magazines – I even had a 3-minute weekly spot on a nationally syndicated radio show called "Something You Should Know."

I started to become famous.

I began speaking to dozens of singles groups and thousands of singles throughout Southern California. I was giving private lessons. I even taught courses for a brief time at Glendale Junior College in Glendale, California.

I began recording talks and new content on the new technology that was available at the time, "cassette tapes," and "VHS video tapes." I was on the threshold of becoming a nationally recognized dating expert. I'm proud to say that I was probably the third one ever to write a "How to" book on attracting women, right after Ovid in 1 BC and of course Eric Weber in 1970.

You have to realize, at the time, there wasn't any competition for dating experts or coaches. In fact, they were unheard of. I'm proud to say I was one of the first.

FURTHER PROOF THE INFORMATION WORKED

Proof my work was valid came when one of the girls I was dating read my book which I penned under the name of Steven Zapman, "How to Attract Men (And Keep Them Interested). You can still find it on Amazon if you look under Steven Zapman, how to attract men. My life was a blur after that, but the next thing I remember is I was married with a child. I did not realize it at the time, but revealed in the book was my source code combined with Kryptonite.

The career of a dating expert is not generally conducive to marriage. My speaking engagements and presentations would cause me to come home late at night. My book tours kept me away from home. To supplement my income, I also provided personal coaching on the side. As fate would have it, various women started calling our house late at night requesting "private lessons."

Shortly thereafter, I heard those four "special" words that cause male sphincters to pucker. My wife said to me, "We need to talk." I'm sure this phenomenon crosses all cultures.

To make a long story very short, I chose marriage, family and a career in commercial real estate over my dating profession. This cut short my blossoming career as an author and dating consultant. For the next several years I sold commercial real estate…

If you want to hear the rest of my story, I posted it at the end of this book.

To be continued(See Epilogue, the rebirth of my life and career)

But enough about me for now. I'm sure you want to get into the "how to" stuff. I saved the best for last, so you can read the rest of my story at the end of this book. My promise now is to show you how to attract women with humor and body language and make them want you.

Next we're going to start with a short experiment, then we'll get into the "attractor factors" or the reasons women are attracted to men so you can learn how to develop those characteristics To Make Women Want You!

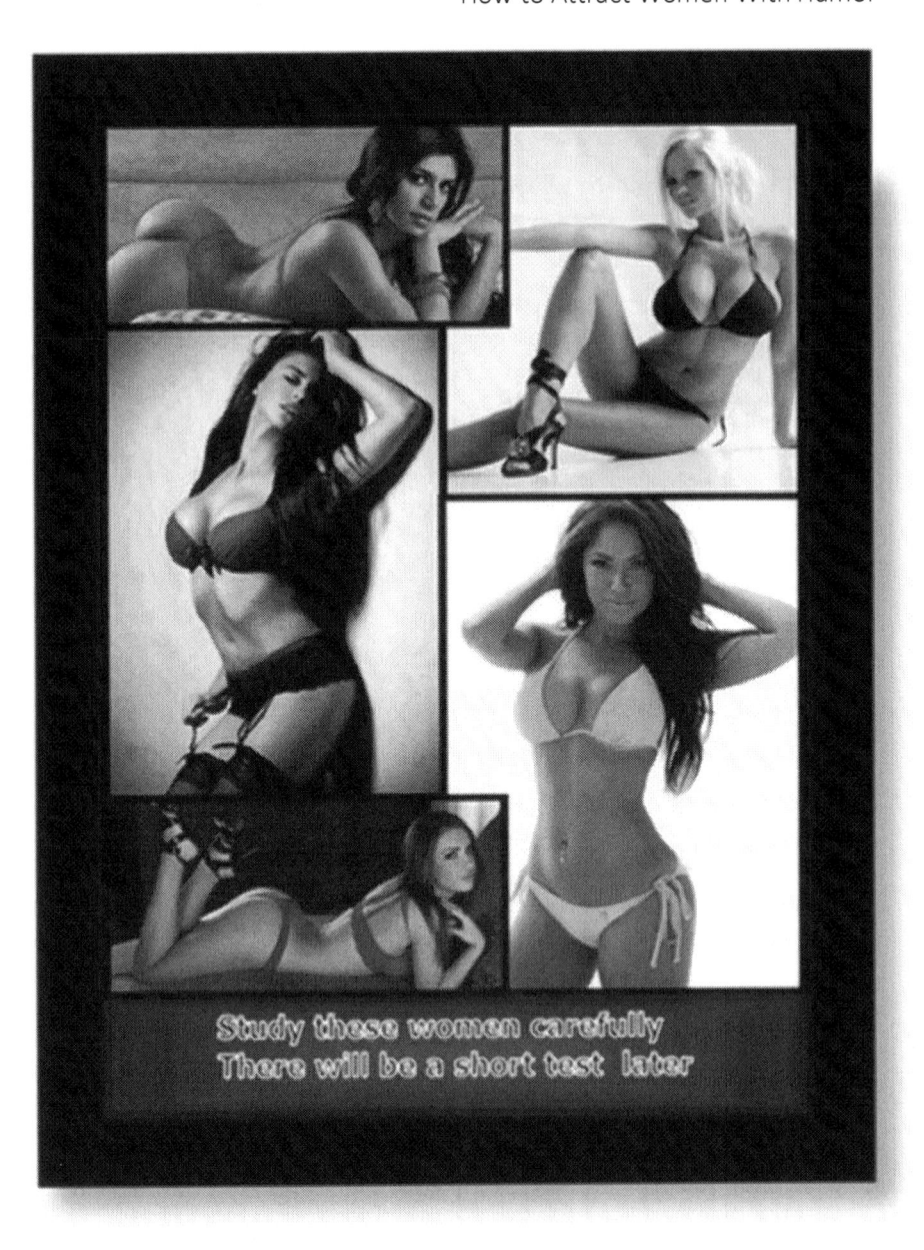

How to Attract Women With Humor

Study these women carefully
There will be a short test later

CHAPTER 4 - THE REASONS WOMEN ARE ATTRACTED TO MEN

THE ATTRACTOR FACTORS THAT MAKE YOU DESIRABLE TO FEMALES

I'm going to let you in on a little secret. Real men want to have as much sex as possible with as many beautiful women that will let them. I know you're probably shocked at this astonishing revelation, but don't be alarmed. It's not your fault, and it's nothing to hide or be ashamed about. In fact, if your ancestors didn't feel the same way, you wouldn't be here.

Chris Rock once said, "A man is basically as faithful as his options."

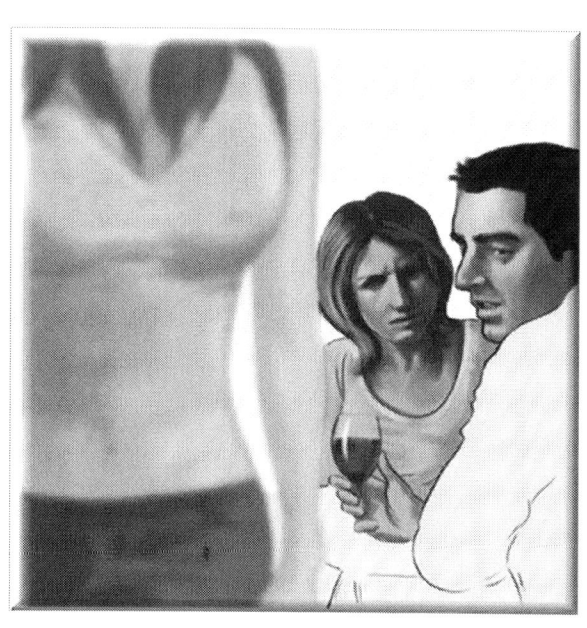

It's important to add that *most* honorable men in a relationship generally restrain themselves from acting on this primal desire mostly out of love and respect for their partner, and to avoid hurting them.

However, that doesn't mean this powerful urge still doesn't exist. To this day learning to control this instinctive impulse tends to be the ultimate male dilemma.

How to Attract Women With Humor

Throughout history, the irresistible urge to have sex with women outside of conventional boundaries has changed history. Kingdoms and dynasties crumbled, nations waged wars, millions of people died, vast fortunes were lost, and Presidents tarnished their legacies, all because of a four-inch magic triangle of mobile real estate.

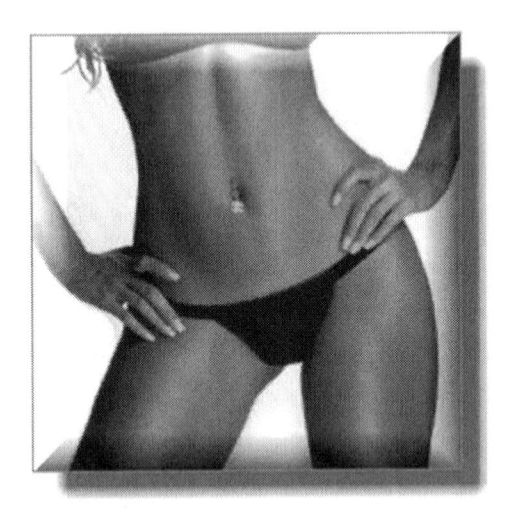

This overpowering urge to have dishonest sex with women still happens every day even at the risk and expense of one losing their career, their family and everything they own, sometimes including one's own life. It defies logic and reason, unless of course you're the one caught in the moment. Then it makes perfectly good sense at the time.

Have you heard of Ashley Madison.com?

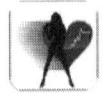

We know that men generally can't control themselves, but guess what? Women are no different in this regard either. Women desire and crave sex too. However, the purpose of this chapter is not only to spotlight the overwhelming force that drives men, but also to reveal the subconscious primal urges and desires that cause women to pursue men for sex.

Understanding and leveraging these reasons will help you to attract women so you can make them want you and to make it easier and more likely for them to have sex with you. Among the many reasons, humor is one of key factors.

Women want men to pursue them for sex. The problem is, too many guys are either too passive and conceal their sexual interest in women, or they act like aggressive idiots and drive them away.

Luckily for you, there is a very cool and natural way to approach and attract women so they become interested in you first, and I'm going to show you how to do it.

There is no doubt that women want to be sexually attractive and desired by men. They are actively looking for those men who have the ability to unlock the code to their natural instinctive desires. This book is going to teach you how to develop those traits and skills that tap into a woman's primal needs and desires. You will become in so many words – simply irresistible.

Man's sex drive is responsible for humans becoming the dominant species on earth. Man's desire to have abundant sex with as many beautiful women as possible is the main reason for practically everything man has ever created or invented since the dawn of humanity.

It's this primal overwhelming urge to merge that motivated our male ancestors to develop and adopt certain traits to mate that are attractive to women. These traits are behaviors and qualities that promote and assist in the survival and growth of the human species.

Humans exist for two main reasons, survival, and reproduction. Men instinctively desire multiple women to mate with in order to produce as many offspring as possible.

Women instinctively choose the highest value men with which they are capable of mating. They are attracted to men who can help them and their offspring survive and thrive, and of course survival in today's society means living in the most safe, comfortable and prosperous lifestyle as possible.

On a primal level, women are generally attracted to men based on the value they can supply to their life. This usually includes status, resources, health, kindness, humor, and other traits necessary to add quality and value to a relationship. These are the primary elements for attraction. There are several other factors as you'll soon find out

I name these traits and characteristics "Attractor Factors." They have evolved and morphed over time, but not as much as you might imagine. They continue to be powerful and irresistible but nonetheless their origins are still primal.

There was a time when the biggest baddest dude in the tribe had the most desirable women nearly all to himself. The ancestral women were attracted to the strongest males because they were the most likely to ensure her and their offspring's survival. This is natural selection as Darwin taught us. Today, resources, status, and adaptability have replaced strength and dominance as the predominant factors.

According to Geoffrey Miller, one of the world's foremost authorities on evolutionary psychology, encoded in a man's DNA is the fear of approaching attractive women, and the fear still exists even after hundreds of thousands of years.

He says that in order for our ancestors to mate with attractive women, they would have to challenge the leader and/ or his associates for the privilege. Often a substantial ass kicking and even death sometimes ensued for the right to mate with the finest women.

This was an incredible revelation to me because it helped me to overcome a fear factor of approaching women that in reality doesn't exist today – well, I suppose it still could depending on where you go to meet women.

Nonetheless, since women are able to procreate only every year or so, she must be very selective with whom she chooses to mate or have sex. Most young men on the other hand, can procreate three to five times a day – so man's motivation is primarily quantity before quality.

A woman's investment in having sex is by far much greater. Her DNA programs her to grow a baby for 9 months then take care of the child for another 18 years or more until it is on his or her own. Nowadays, that age often reaches 30 or longer. Perhaps you know someone like this.

For these reasons, psychologically it's generally much easier for men to have sex than women. This is a perfect example of how our evolutionary history has created certain irresistible behaviors between the sexes.

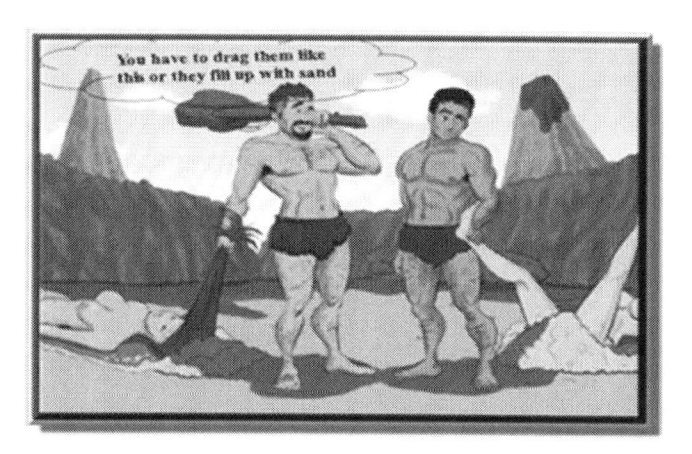

Back in the day, it was so easy any caveman could do it – and he usually did, whenever he wanted to.

However, over time as humans

evolved and became more civilized, women started demanding more control over with whom they chose to have sex. Unfortunately, cameras or keyboards weren't around to document when and how women started changing men's behavior to make sex more consensual.

It's my opinion that women, by either causing men extreme bowel discomfort when "inadvertently" contaminating their food, or "accidently" using their teeth when servicing them, finally got across their point. Eventually men had to start compromising more by wooing and courting women to avoid future "mishaps."

The need to level the playing field and a quid pro quo exchange forced men to start developing skills and traits to exchange for sexual favors, with romantic gestures being a part of them. I would be willing to bet the need to modify men's behavior in exchange for sex was the first women's rights cause and rally that took place.

It was most likely the first agenda on the list of many other women's demands to follow. One could say it was the beginning of women's equal rights and how the "women's movement" (in more ways than one) acquired them.

Intelligence and adaptability began replacing strength and dominance as the primary attractor factors. Men started developing more skills that eventually led to the creation of math, science, history and unraveling the mysteries of life.

Musicians, writers, comics, and artists also evolved from this primordial soup of skill sets because these talents were a sign of intelligence, adaptability, and creativity.

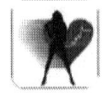

The desire for more sex continued to motivate men to develop aptitudes that brought value and resources to the tribe and marketplace. These aptitudes or fitness indicators aroused the desire and passion in women, so women would want to have sex with the men who were the most worthy because they could bring the value and resources to them and their offspring.

Actors and rock stars train to develop skill sets of attraction and so can you. Humor is another major attractor factor because of the pleasurable endorphins it releases in our brains. You can train yourself to become more humorous too!

At the top of this chapter, I posted a picture of five sexy women. If you're listening on the audiobook, I want you to take a minute to visualize five incredibly gorgeous, voluptuous sexy young women in their mid to late twenties. They are scantily dressed in skimpy bathing suits in various seductive poses.

One is posing laying down, another on her hands and knees, you get the picture. They are all looking at you with lust in their eyes, like they must have you, right here and right now.

Have those images and thoughts marinated in your brain yet?

Now, I want you to answer quickly these questions:

- *Did that exercise alter your consciousness?*

- *What did those thoughts make you feel?*

- *How did it change your focus?*

- *What did it make you want to do?*

The purpose of this simple exercise is give you a firsthand account how at a primal level the sensation of irresistible attraction automatically affects our brain chemistry. It ignites our pleasure centers that start a chain reaction of signals and messages to the rest of our body.

It's as if our brain was a conductor that singlehandedly cued a symphony of music using our body parts as instruments. It starts with enlarged pupils, to an increased heart rate, to sweat gland and hormonal production, which then start to produce the crescendo of pleasurable feelings and the beginning states of arousal.

These visual cues are prime examples of the "Attractor Factors" and "Traits to Mate" that women exhibit which attracts men irresistibly to them, even by the mere sight of pictures.

Neuroscientists Sai Goddam and Ogi Ogas analyzed a billion web searches, a million Web sites, a million erotic videos, a million erotic stories, millions of personal ads, and tens of thousands of digitized romance novels to determine what really turns people on.

In their book "[A Billion Wicked Thoughts]()," their groundbreaking findings profoundly alter the way you think about the sexual relationships of women and men...

One determination was that men are aroused more by visual cues. A man looks at a woman searching for sexual stimuli like a jeweler looks for perfection in a flawless gem. Visual cues convey information about a woman's health, fertility, and youth.

Women are aroused more by psychological cues. A woman looks at a man much like a detective would a suspected criminal who is about to commit another crime. The visual cues a woman looks for are status, resources, commitment, kindness, stability, and competence.

The example they used for men is the cartoon character Elmer Fudd, who continues to hunt for rabbits no matter how many times Bugs Bunny fools him or leads him on. Elmer has a one-track mind and nothing else matters than to shoot a silly wabbit.

The example they used for women is Ms. Marple, the famous woman detective in Agatha Christies' mystery novels. Based on her vast experience and intuition, she closely examines and evaluates a male suspect to determine whether he's innocent or guilty.

The purpose of this book is to demonstrate that women are also prone to these sensations of irresistible attraction and sexual arousal, except their criteria for attraction to certain men are very different in many respects from the ones that men experience for women.

According to a report in Medscape.com, Women prefer erotic stimulation with a story line and erotic mood. Dating expert Lance Mason calls it "male cleavage." If you need proof, look at the success of "50 Shades of Gray."

Attraction is not a choice (an awesome quote from another top dating guru, David DeAngelo). These are natural biological reactions embedded in our DNA developed over tens of thousands of years. Just as men have these responses to attractive women, so do women have similar reactions when they observe men with certain masculine traits.

We often think of the male as competing with other males for the prize of mating with the most desirable female, but women, of course, also compete for the opportunity to mate and live with the male who has the most desirable traits.

You'll discover what those masculine traits are and how you can couple them with humor to develop and use them to your advantage. I'm happy to report that some of you guys will be very relieved to know that looks aren't at the top of the list of attractor factors for women. I'm just saying…

Have you ever wondered why you are attracted to a certain type of woman, while other men may not be? The same thing happens for women.

Some women can find one man extraordinarily appealing while her friends would totally rule him out. Many people would attribute this attraction to "chemistry."

THE SCENT OF A WOMAN

There definitely is some body chemistry going on – like pheromones, from the scent of a woman – and a man. This happens at an instinctive and involuntary level. Research performed on females by scientist F. Bryant Furlow in 1996 shows that women on a subconscious level prefer men whose genes are the least similar to their own.

Her brain and advanced ability to smell is able to decode instinctually the state of a man's immune system within 3 seconds of meeting. If it's complementary to or stronger than her own immune system, she may find that man very attractive, or strangely magnetic. If her immune system is stronger than his is, she is likely to find him less attractive.

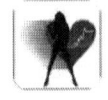

By choosing a mate whose molecules (and thus their pheromones or scent) is complementary or stronger than their own, males and females are ensuring that their offspring will have a wider variety of molecules, or DNA. This allows us to be better able to identify a larger array of invaders (bacteria and viruses) and thus create a better immune system to promote survival for our offspring.

But wait – there's more to why we find ourselves attracted to certain types of women. Another significant reason is due to the combination of impressions and things we have seen, heard, smelled, tasted, and touched throughout our formative years of growing up.

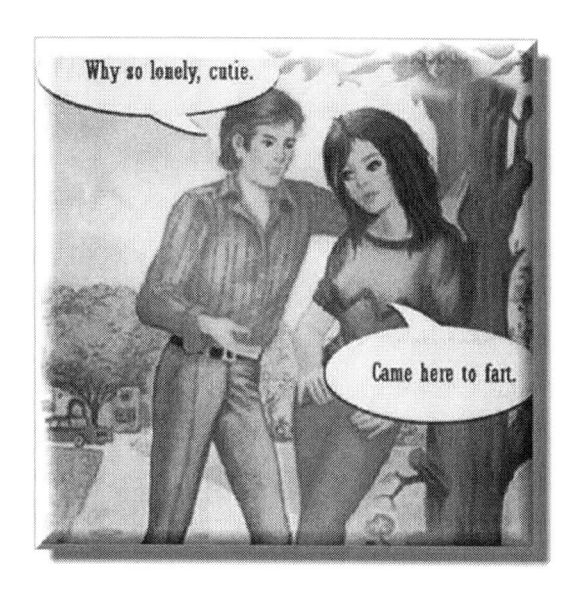

HEROES AND VILLAINS

A number of things contribute to the development of our attitudes toward things or people one may perceive as desirable or undesirable. Our mothers and fathers, our friends and associates, books we read, television programs and movies we saw, heroes and villains we have admired and abhorred, the sex symbol of the year, etc. all contribute to what we find attractive or unattractive.

If, in the past, we have associated certain things with pleasure and enjoyment, we will most likely have a favorable disposition toward similar objects or people in the present and in the future. We associate them with pleasure, and we will become attracted to them.

Likewise, if the experience was not pleasurable, we may have just the opposite attitude toward it; one of disdain or disapproval and something we want to avoid.

For example, if a young girl had a dentist who had a beard and made her cry when he worked on her teeth, that experience could shape her opinion of men with beards for the rest of her life. She may not like men with beards.

On the other hand, if her grandfather had a beard and was kind and loving to her, she would likely be more favorable with men having them.

The major exception to this rule is our parents. Since they generally were our first contact with the world and the primary providers of our survival, their treatment of us is what we associate with love and affection – even if they treated us terribly or lovingly.

This is the reason why it is common that women usually end up marrying or being attracted to men who resemble their father. She associates her father with pleasurable and loving experiences like security, emotional well being, comfort, and even food. Therefore, she will often seek a man similar in appearance and personality.

Studies show that most women are more likely to pair up with men whose behavior and bone structure are similar to their own father. The phenomenon is "sexual imprinting," and this study suggests that the faces and behavior we find appealing as adults are determined in childhood.

Even in the event her father was a dysfunctional alcoholic and did not provide any emotional security or loving when she was young, she would still find these types of men attractive because her brain imprinted that type of behavior as being loving and affectionate.

At the beginning of her life, there was no point of reference to measure or compare with proper child rearing. At that age, one is unable to distinguish between acceptable or unacceptable behavior.

Fortunately, some women come to realize what a healthy relationship consists of and are able to overcome the powerful but dysfunctional attraction of an unhealthy relationship. By the way, sexual imprinting affects men the same way.

LOVE THYSELF AS THY NEIGHBOR?

A multitude of studies has shown that we are attracted to people who resemble ourselves, especially if we have a high level of self-esteem. So don't be surprised if you find yourself attracted to another person who looks and acts just as you do.

Another factor that determines to whom we are attracted are our relationships with ex-girlfriends and past women we have been involved with or attracted. How many guys do you know who break up with a woman only to find themselves immediately involved with another one who is a spitting image of her? Think about yourself and the women to whom you've been attracted.

This also includes long lost loves, even puppy love or junior high school girl friends you liked. Deep in your subconscious mind are the memories and images connected with the pleasure you felt when you were with those girls or women. You don't forget them and they will determine to a large degree what you find attractive now and into the future.

FRIENDS AND FAMILY

Your friends and family also have an influence on whom or what you determine is desirable or undesirable. This conditioning takes place throughout your lifetime. If you have a closely-knit family and they have put a great deal of emphasis on marrying within your race or religion, then oftentimes you will find someone who fits that ideal.

In addition, since most people seek the approval of their friends, they will often influence who you should become attracted to merely through peer pressure.

The media also portrays what is "supposed" to be desirable and attractive. This is of course always transitory. If you remember the James Bond movie "Dr. No" where Ursula Andress comes out of the water dripping wet with her hard nipples showing through her skimpy bathing suit – that made any woman who resembled her extremely desirable at the time.

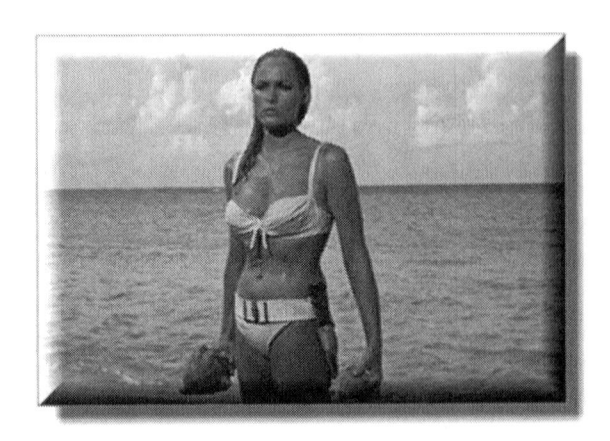

These same principles apply to women. Therefore, not only do earlier experiences dictate what a woman perceives as attractive, so do current sex symbols like Brad Pitt or George Clooney. If you have the fortune of resembling either of these two, probably many women will find you very attractive.

So you see, even before a woman (or women) sets her eyes upon you, she already has a preconceived notion about what she deems as attractive or unattractive. The computers in our brains are remarkably fast at making almost instantaneous calculations concerning the desirability of another person.

All of our past and present experiences are immediately tabulated; experiences concerning race, religion, appearance, mood, age, size, shape, posture, sound, smell, education, etc. and whirr, click click, buzzzz-out comes the answer; yes, no or maybe (until more information is fed into the computer).

In 2005, Malcolm Gladwell wrote a book called "Blink." Blink is about how we think about choices that seem to be made in an instant — in the blink of an eye. These choices actually aren't as simple as they seem, and those instantaneous decisions are often impossible to explain to others.

He studied "Speed Daters" where men and women spent 3 minutes talking to each other to determine if there was an attraction between them. Before he analyzed the data, he asked the women what characteristics they were looking for in a man or men.

What he discovered was that the women were attracted to certain men based upon split second decisions. Ultimately, he determined that they did not match the characteristics of the type of men they thought they were looking for.

The conclusion? We have, as human beings, a storytelling problem. We're a bit too quick to come up with explanations for things which we really don't have an explanation. So in most cases, women are not always attracted to what they think they want in a man – and that goes for men as well.

Our emotional brain tells us we should like a certain type of trait in a mate, and that may be true at that moment in time – however short-lived it may be. However, the primal limbic part of our brain tends to default back to what our ancestors found attractive for survival and healthy offspring – the attractor factors I've previously mentioned.

I'm sure you've heard countless women say they want a warm sensitive guy that can cry, that treats them right and does all these nice things for them. Then they lose respect for him, they become too demanding; and the next thing you know you find out they start screwing the first bad boy they meet.

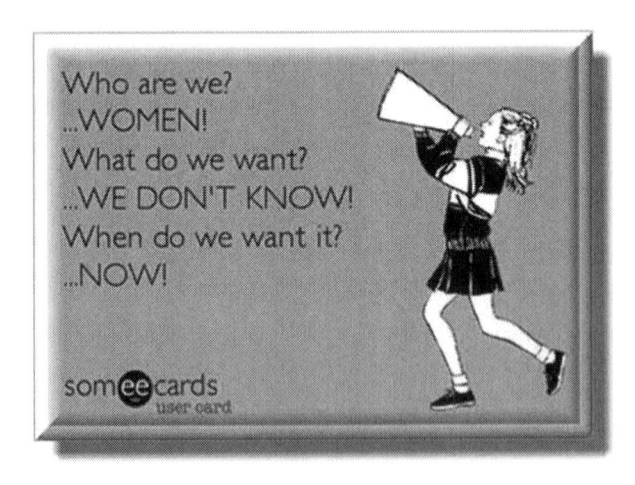

> Who are we?
> ...WOMEN!
> What do we want?
> ...WE DON'T KNOW!
> When do we want it?
> ...NOW!
>
> someecards user card

Sigmund Freud asked that immortal question over a hundred years ago, "What does a woman want?"

Who are we? Women! What do we want? We don't know! When do we want it? Now!

I guess this shows that even the women themselves don't even know!"

The reasons for attraction are obviously numerous and sometimes undetectable; nevertheless, the subconscious mind thinks it knows in advance what to look for, but it isn't always right.

Rutgers University anthropologist Helen Fisher summarizes one of the best explanations I've ever heard on the reasons for love and attraction in humans:

> *"The human body is such a finely tuned attraction seeking machine. It takes only one second to decide intuitively whether someone's physically hot or not. When it comes to love (or lust, as the case may be), men and women unconsciously know what they like when they see it.*
>
> *To help ensure that the good ones don't get away, our bodies produce a variety of physical signs of attraction that grab our attention and direct it toward the object of our desire. When those physiological mechanisms kick in, even a brief glimpse of a crush can leave us short of breath and dazed. "*

One's subconscious preselection thus involves the entire mental makeup of a person. His or her ideal notion of what is attractive can involve a number of factors as we have seen.

Therefore, the number of possibilities or combinations of what is attractive to one woman and not another largely depends on each woman's personal history and experiences. The purpose of this book is to show you how to increase your attractiveness to the most women and cover as many bases as possible.

If you want to enjoy life's ultimate pleasure of falling in love and being in love, then you can have it if you are willing to take the necessary steps I'm about to share. Having a passionate romantic sex life with someone you truly love and want to share your life with, is in my opinion life's ultimate experience.

I can't think of a more important decision that you will ever make regarding your happiness than with whom you choose to share your life. Finding a quality woman all begins with first meeting her, and in order to meet her, you'll need to know how to approach and cause her to become attracted and interested in you.

CHAPTER 5 - HOW TO MASTER NON-VERBAL COMMUNICATION

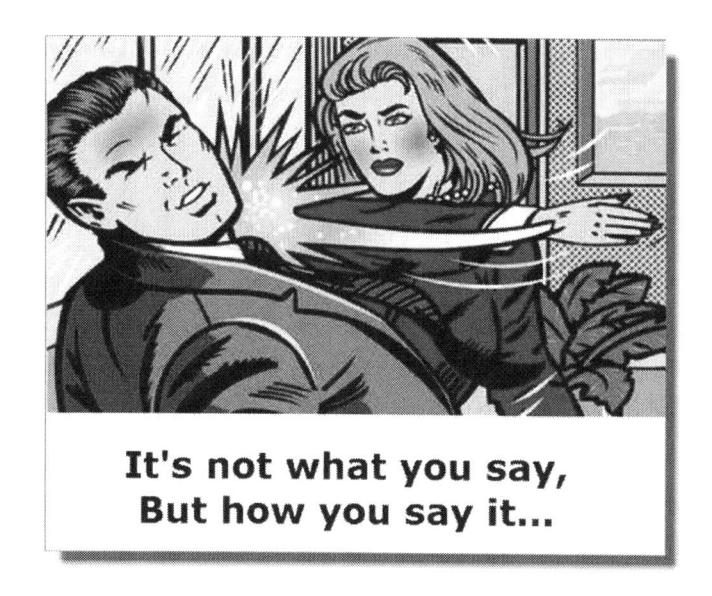

It's not what you say, But how you say it...

It's not what you say but how you say it that commands interest and attention.

Dr. Joyce Brothers writes, "Less than 10 percent of what we communicate to other people is conveyed by words. About 35 percent comes from the way we speak, the tone of voice, whether we mumble or shout. The other 55 percent comes from body movements and facial expressions."

Scientists sometimes divide the study of nonverbal communication into three areas: "Kinesics" (facial expressions and body language), "Proxemics" (the use of space), and "Para language" (voice quality of your delivery).

We express a great deal of our personality in non-verbal ways. Too many of us hide our best side because of our inability to speak with emotion or use our body language properly. Evangelists and politicians are experts at this. They know how to stimulate, excite, and command the attention from their audiences.

Have you ever heard or seen the late President John F. Kennedy say, "Ask not what your country can do for you, but what you can do for your country!" It comes across as commanding and forceful. The late Reverend Dr. Martin Luther King, Jr., was also a master of public speaking. "I've been to the mountaintop, and I've looked over and I've seen the Promised Land!"

These examples demonstrate the effect that proper usage of body language and delivery can have when trying to attract attention and interest. You can model the techniques and styles of the best you wish to emulate to suit your own needs and make yourself a more interesting and exciting person.

5.1 KINESICS (BODY LANGUAGE)

If you really want to be attractive to women and command more respect from everyone, then you must start practicing and mastering masculine body language today – and use it everywhere you go. You MUST make this promise to yourself right now because mastering masculine body language is one of the easiest things you can do to improve your life.

From this day on, you need to be aware of what kind of person you're broadcasting to the world. Your body language is the first thing everyone (especially women) recognizes about you, and it defines who you are to anyone who sees you for the first time.

Masculine Body Language is one of the most important tools you have and probably the easiest to develop of all the Attractor Factors. The way you use your body really does tell a lot about you. It tells you how you are feeling about yourself, how you feel about others, and how others feel about you.

As an experiment to prove this, cut somebody off on the freeway and closely observe their hands and facial expressions. You probably won't be able to hear them, but their message will be clear. Everyone who is able uses their body consciously and unconsciously to communicate messages non-verbally.

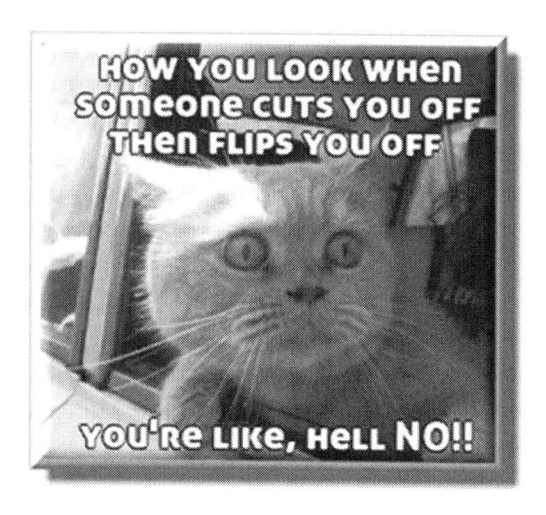

It isn't always necessary for others to tell us what they are thinking or feeling. We can often sense it merely by observing their body. Of course, we can't always be correct when interpreting other people's body language, but the majority of times we can make accurate interpretations by using our intuition, or what famous psychologist Dr. Theodore Reik calls a "third ear."

Through years of experience and conditioning, he says that people are actually able to interpret a meaning from our body movements without even realizing it.

> *"Muscular twitching in the face or hands and movements of the eyes speak to us as well as words. No small power of communication is contained in a glance, a person's bearing, a bodily movement, a special way of breathing ...There are variations in tone, pauses and shifted accentuation so slight that they never reach the limits of conscious observation, which nevertheless betray a great deal to us about a person."*

Even though we may not always realize it, we respond to other people's body movements or "cues" just as they respond to ours. These cues include a variety of postures, facial expressions, gestures, touches, eye movements and voice patterns that when used properly and in the right combinations can either attract or repel people.

You want to avoid nervous movements at all costs. This includes facial twitching, nervous movements of your face, arms, legs, hands, and feet. Tapping your toes or strumming your hands on the desk shows stress, and that translates to lack of confidence.

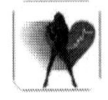

If you feel nervous – you'll make her feel nervous. If you're relaxed, everyone around you will tend to be more relaxed. You will tend to react to the body language of others around you. If you are the one to display the most confidence in the group, others will model your behavior. The name for this act is shaping.

Many of these movements are involuntary and depend on your attitude and self-image at the time. Now that you are aware of the negative "cues" and "signals"; you can consciously replace them with the positive ones to enhance your appeal and make those around you feel more comfortable and welcoming.

Your eyes, face, arms, legs, hands, and entire posture can be an asset or a liability when communicating depending upon how you use them. Not only does it cause others to treat you with more respect when you use them effectively, you will also feel it internally. Employing effective body language will in turn make you feel and act more masculine.

WALKING, STANDING AND SITTING

How do you tell the most powerful person in the room? It's how they carry them self - so if you want to be noticed - you will need to know how to carry yourself, and play the part of the masculine alpha male.

How you walk, stand and sit will absolutely determine how women will react to you. In fact, everyone's perception of you is highly dependent upon your facial expressions and the way you move your body.

Just like most men can't help but look at a woman's cleavage; most women can't help but keep their eyes off a confident man who carries himself well. From this day forward, you must consistently start using dominant, masculine body language if you want to be attractive to women. This includes how you stand, sit, gesture, and walk into and out of a room or walk to wherever it is you're going.

Become aware of every movement you make and make the mastery of your movements a part of your lifestyle. Wherever you go, you should live out these masculine movements until they become natural and a part of you. Your body language will be the first chance women will have to judge who you are.

The first lesson starts with an accurate, erect posture. The best way to practice the ideal posture is to stand in front of a mirror, and imagine that a hook is suspending you at the top of your sternum. Your back should be straight and your shoulders slightly back with your arms hanging naturally at your side. In fact, it's the quickest way to make it look like you've lost 10 pounds when you do this.

When you first enter a crowded room, take a deep breath, stand at the entrance tall and erect for a few moments and scope out the room. Determine where it is you want to go.

Walk in with just a hint of attitude – as if you have big balls – as if you just finished 50 pushups and your arms are huge. Make it appear as natural as possible. Practice in the mirror until you have your own confident style and realize this is the new you. This is how you're going to carry yourself from now on, even when you get up to go to the bathroom in the middle of the night.

When you walk, it's important to walk slowly and purposefully with a measured rhythm. Walk with your shoulders back, your hands slightly clenched, and let your arms swing naturally. Walk like you own the place. Take up room when you walk and tilt your head slightly upwards with a relaxed face. Look forward and not at the ground

How to Attract Women With Humor

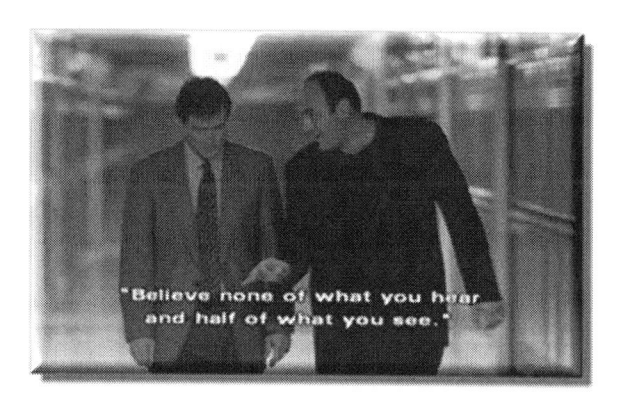

When you walk, take long, deliberate confident strides. Put your heel down first, swing your arms naturally, and walk with a sense of purpose. Imagine Tony Soprano walking into a meeting with his associates, or Dewayne Johnson (The Rock) walking into the ring. They ooze confidence and you can sense their power merely by the way they walk.

When you're standing, it's important that you put all your weight on one leg with your shoulders slightly back. It doesn't matter which one – whichever one makes you feel more comfortable. You'll look much more confident, cool, and relaxed when you do. Try different standing postures in the mirror and you'll see that this one is by far the best.

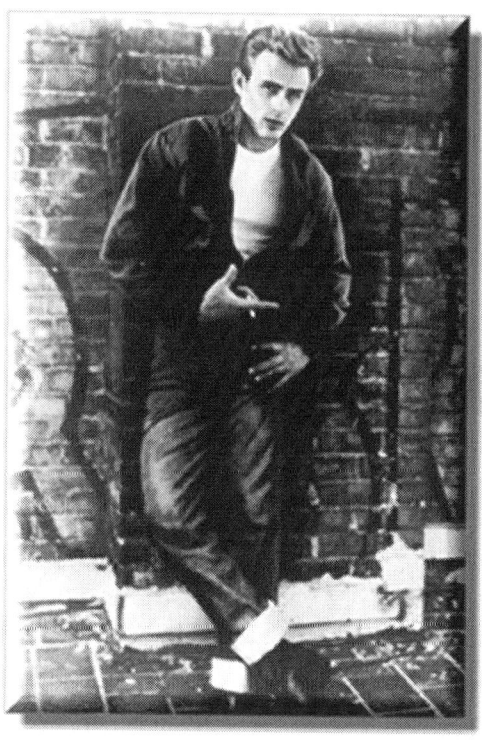

When you sit down, don't plop down in the chair; sit down slowly with grace and ease. Show some coordination, core strength, and class. Imagine how James Bond would sit down. The same thing goes for standing up. Stand up slowly by using your core, it shows strength and stability. Don't lean on things or pull yourself up with something nearby.

Practice all these movements in the mirror until you get them down to perfection. Michael Jackson didn't perfect the moonwalk in one try. Practice them when you get up to walk to the bathroom in the middle of the night. Practice them when you sit down at your computer or at the dinner table.

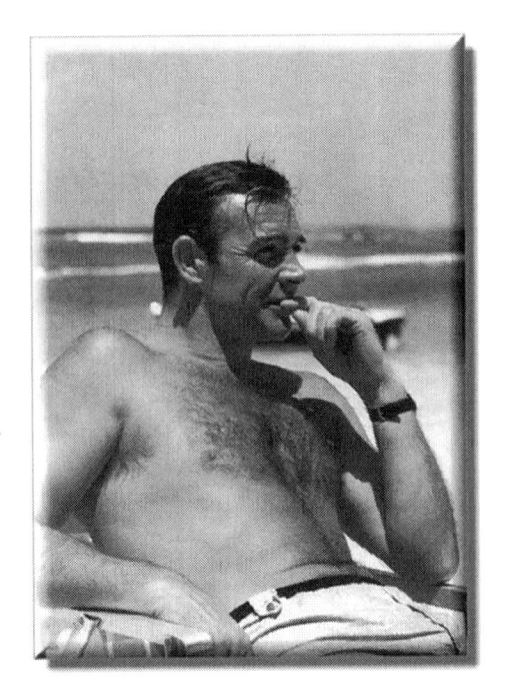

Especially practice them every single time you go out in public and watch your reflection in windows so you can adjust accordingly. You will immediately begin to see how others start to notice and regard you more. When this starts to happen, it will give you a boost of self-confidence to motivate you to master masculine body language with every single move you make.

EYES

Scientists have discovered at least four major reasons why it is important to maintain eye contact:

- It is an indicator of how we feel about ourselves.

- It lets others know that a communication channel is open.

- It communicates intimate feelings.

- It is a multiplier of sentiments.

In order to have more self-confidence you should make more eye contact because studies have shown that people who feel good about themselves use more eye contact. "The amount of eye contact engaged in by subjects has been found to correlate positively with their self reports of liking." says Dr. Zick Rubin.

Second, eye contact also lets others know that we wish to have a meeting of the minds. "Eye contact serves as a mutually understood signal that communication is open between two people."

Third, your eyes serve to express your innermost feelings. They can have a tremendous amount of impact on the words or feelings you are trying to express. Try to picture how effective or meaningful the words "I love you" are without intimate eye contact - Not very much, unless you are blind.

Last, looking at each other eye to eye adds a significant increase to the thrust and impact of your words, whether they are cheerful or angry.

Your eyes can have a very overpowering effect when dealing with women. Learn to flirt with them, not only when looking directly in her eyes. You should also allow yourself to gaze at her hair, ears, and nose; linger on her lips, and shoulders.

You should avoid staring at her tits and ass until you have mutually established a sexual connection or you may scare them off. Your approach in this regard needs to be gradual and mutual, as you'll discover later.

Timing is everything when you flirt with your eyes, and you want to make sure that the conversation, location and mood is primed for it. Many studies have shown that when we like what we see or when we experience something very pleasurable, the size of our pupils increase.

Unconsciously, this transmits a seductive or loving message to the other person and makes us more appealing.

Centuries ago, women used to put belladonna in their eyes to create this effect artificially. Today, we know that photographers touch up their photographs with ink instead of belladonna to produce the same effect. A dimly lighted room, candlelight, fireplace, or moonlight will produce the same effect for your own purposes.

According to Desmond Morris there is a slight increase in tear production when our emotions run high which tends to make our eyes "sparkle." This also enhances your appeal to an onlooker and when combined with the pupil dilation it gives the effect of a person in love.

A very effective way of using your eyes is to hold a glance slightly longer than you usually would, as if you were in a trance. Slowly blink your eyes while doing this and a woman will wonder what you have on your mind. She will no doubt feel attraction for, or at least to what you are thinking.

How to Attract Women With Humor

I've described in detail below five different very effective techniques you can use with your eyes to create strong attraction:

1. Eye Triangulation - One of the more powerful techniques for instant attraction is eye triangulation. When you're interested in a woman and she is telling you something very important, gaze into her left eye for a few seconds, then move to her right one for a few more, then down to her mouth for about 4 seconds. Slowly do this a few times and she will become mesmerized.

2. Shaping Stare – At the right moment, you want to look at her as if she's the only one in the room. Sean Connery can seduce women with his hypnotic eye contact alone. Look deeply into her eyes, and imagine that you're reading her mind and it's telling you that she can't wait to sleep with you. Slowly lick your lips and fondle your glass for further effect. Your seductive look will communicate back to her that very message.

3. False Affront followed by The Macho Man Squint - You've been teasing her all night, so eventually she'll try to get back at you. Wait until she teases or challenges you about something and then give her the bad boy Macho Man Squint as if you're offended. It's the one where Clint Eastwood says, "Go ahead, make my day."

Give her the look for about three seconds as if you're insulted. She may get uneasy or embarrassed when she thinks you're offended. Wait as long as possible, then go ahead and laugh it off together. The timing is critical on this one.

This procedure is so effective because the humor releases the built up tension, much as an apology releases tension after a fight, and then you know how this usually results in great makeup sex.

This type of dynamic combined with the tug of war principle make relationships exciting, especially in the early stages.

A great illustration of the psychology behind this power is demonstrated in the bar scene in Goodfellas where Joe Pesci asks Ray Liotta "I'm funny how, I mean funny like I'm a clown?"

Watch how the tension builds, and then notice how you feel when it is released. This is a prime example of the primal emotion of excitement, attraction and power you experience under these circumstances.

4. Fake Pass - Hold your gaze on her while she's involved in doing something away from you, like driving or reading. Wait until she finally looks back at you and asks, "What?" – You smile, then start to say something, then say "oh nothing." This will drive her crazy and she will playfully insist on you telling her. Keep telling her that you weren't going to say anything.

Hold out as long as you can, then finally say, "You've got some spinach in your teeth." When she looks in the mirror and finds out you were just teasing her, she will start cracking up and probably try to punch your arm playfully. She will be embarrassed, amused and flattered all at the same time.

5. Forward Pass – The same as the Fake Pass, but instead of teasing her when she asks "What?" you smile and tell her that you just like looking at her and tell her how much she turns you on. You just scored some major points.

I have one last note on eye contact. Your blink rate is very important. When you are engaged in heavy eye contact, try to blink as little as possible, and when you have to, do it very slowly. This helps to increase seduction.

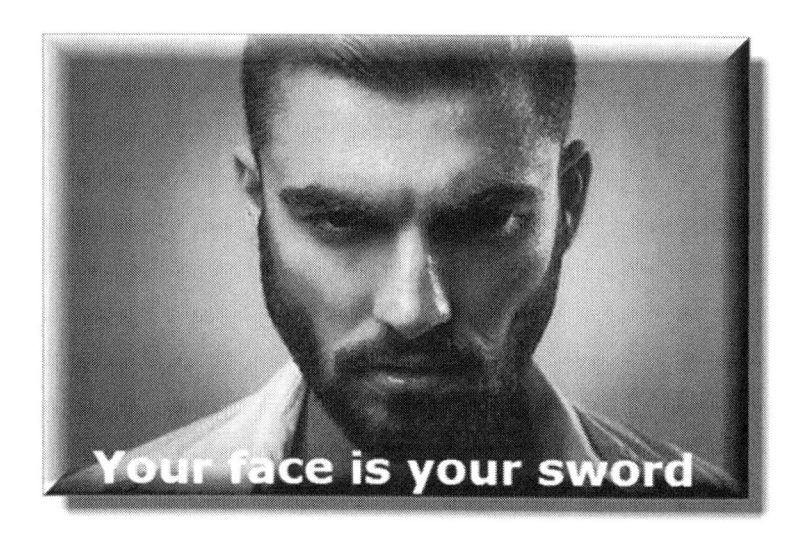

FACE AND HEAD

YOUR FACE IS YOUR SWORD.

Your face is another demonstrative tool you have at your disposal to express interest or sentiments, and is without a doubt the most expressive part of your body. However, as I explained earlier, your attitude and self-image have a great deal to do with your facial expressions, and your true feelings and your face can often betray lack of self-confidence.

Even though you may try hard to make your face look attractive and appealing, part of the truth nevertheless shows through. According to Julius Fast in his book *The Body Language of Sex, Power and Aggression*, slow motion pictures were taken to study peoples' faces when they tried to cover up their emotions, and momentary flickers showed the emotions these people really felt; feelings like disgust, anger, boredom and annoyance.

Mr. Fast notes, "These are flickers that pass so rapidly that the untrained eye cannot sort them out. But a part of your brain does observe them and record them, even though it all happens too fast for conscious recognition."

These records are fed into the storage and computer processing center of our brain, and we react to the hidden message." This is further justification for working on your attitude and self-image to demonstrate more confidence and charisma. Giving yourself a pep talk prior to important encounters is also extremely helpful.

Your face can signal the entire gamut of emotions ranging from frustration, sadness and anger, to contentment, happiness and ecstasy. A face that looks cheerful, alert and excited attracts us strongly, while a face that looks angry or grumpy will probably have the opposite effect.

One of the easiest and best ways to use your face to your advantage is to learn to relax your jaw. Dating expert Lance Mason first brought this concept to my attention and it truly is a breakthrough technique. Women are extremely adept at reading your facial expressions, and one of the most telling signs of being nervous is a tense jaw.

You should check yourself out in a mirror and notice the difference it makes in your demeanor when you practice this. Your smile becomes more natural, and it's much easier to give sly, sexy grins. Porn starts use it all the time and Bill Clinton is a master at it.

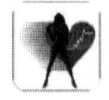

How to Attract Women With Humor

It can also help to relax your body and have the effect of changing your whole mood. It might feel a little odd at first, but this one technique will make a huge difference in your presentation. Try relaxing your jaw when you want to relax.

Your facial expressions play a very important part when listening to others talk. They serve as a mirror reflecting your interest in what the other person is saying. If you simply stare with a deadpan expression at another person while they are talking, they will soon become uneasy and look for a way out of the conversation.

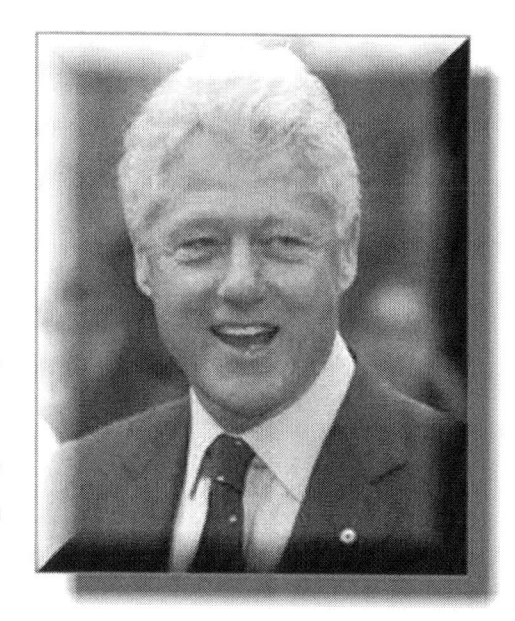

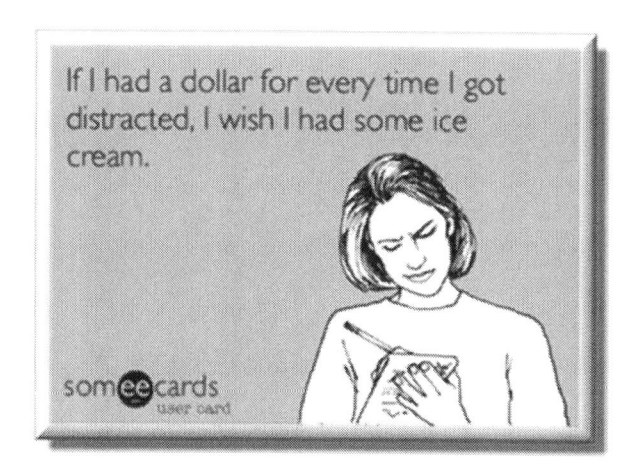

You are actually telling the other person that they are boring you, or that you would rather be somewhere else. In addition, if you speak with a look of disinterest on your face, you'll come across as dull and uninteresting. Allow your face to express sincere interest or show appropriate emotions when talking or listening.

You may use all sorts of facial expressions to show that you're listening: smiling, frowning, looking surprised, looking disgusted, looking shocked, etc. Try to feel what she is saying and don't be afraid to show concern. This is equivalent to letting her know you're truly interested and are paying close attention to what she's saying.

A nod of the head also indicates an interest in what she's saying. It doesn't necessarily mean that you agree with her, but it does give her the message that you're listening carefully and attentively.

A forward lean in addition to nodding is an even more effective way of letting her know how interested you are. Apart from your eyes, your smile is probably your second most important facial asset.

A subtle smile lets her know that you like what you're seeing, that you like the way you're feeling, or a combination of both. It's important not to smile too broadly or too much, remember the Alpha Male rules; be very sparing with your approval.

ARMS

You can use your arms to either welcome or embrace others, or fold them in front of you to create a barrier and demonstrate weakness, defensiveness, or resistance. Of course, you should take context and other body language cues into consideration. It could also mean someone is cold or it's just a way for them to feel comfortable.

How to Attract Women With Humor

You should know that studies have shown that your credibility is substantially reduced and others will think you're not approachable when you cross your arms. You should avoid it if you want to influence someone to your way of thinking.

You should also avoid what the broken zipper position. It's the same position men take in a line at soup kitchens or when receiving social security benefits. It reveals dejected, vulnerable feelings. Adolf Hitler used it regularly in public to mask the sexual inadequacy he felt because of having only one testicle.

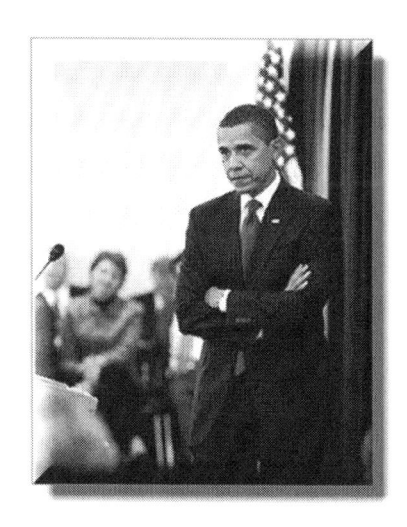

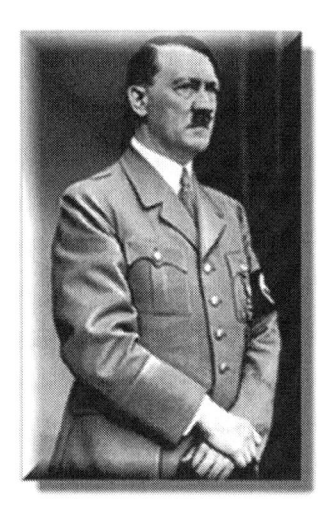

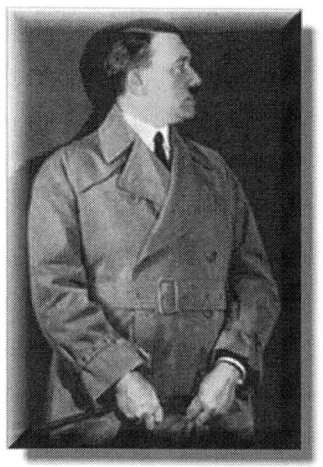

85 | Page

How to Attract Women With Humor

Politicians, royalty, celebrities, and TV personalities disguise their nervousness by using the cufflink fix. This is a trademark of Johnny Carson and he used it whenever one of his jokes bombed. Prince Charles uses it to give himself a feeling of security anytime he walks across an open space in full view of anyone.

The confident masculine man uses his arms to create space around himself, for example when he sits on a sofa; he extends his arms to carve out his territory. He does it to make him feel comfortable and in control.

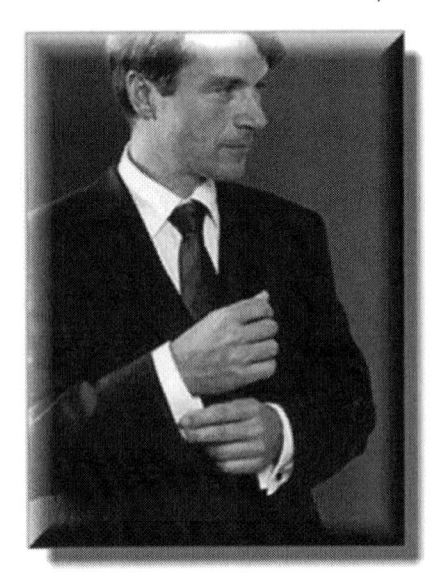

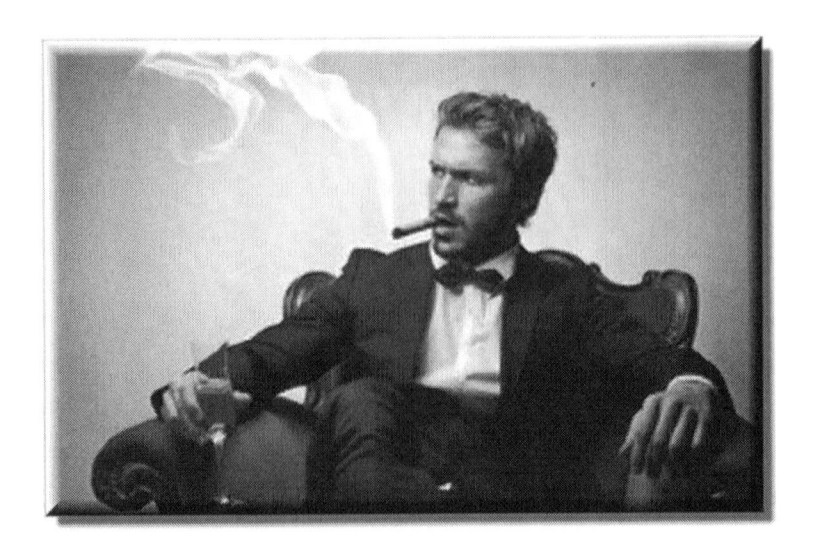

86 | Page

Of course you can also use them to welcome an embrace from a woman. When you have determined that a woman's body language is welcoming, then with your newfound confidence, you can hold out your arms and you can be sure that she will welcome your invitation.

When you do give her a hug, make sure it's masculine where there's full body contact lasting at least 3 seconds. I'm not talking about a bear hug. You want to embrace enough to feel your hips firmly touching while you smell the perfume on her neck. You should put your left hand on her waist and use your right arm around her shoulder to bring her into you.

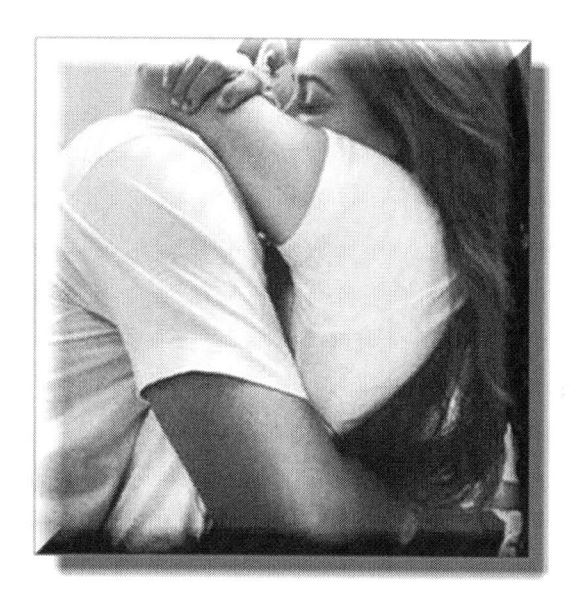

When you release, finish the hug with direct eye contact and the sexy grin you've been practicing in the mirror. Make it last a few more seconds. Make it seem like you have a secret just between you.

LEGS

In the walking section, I covered how to use your legs when walking. When sitting, you can cross them when you're able to use your arms to create space, but crossing your legs and holding them tightly together when you don't have room to extend your arms does not send out confident masculine signals.

If you're sitting at a bar or in a room and you want to show interest or welcome a woman into your world, open your legs like a V wide enough to envelop her presence. The stronger a connection you're able to establish, the wider you can open them as she moves closer to you.

You don't usually notice these strong body language signals at the conscious level. You should avoid closing your legs tightly or point them away from her. She will think you are disinterested.

When observing the body language of women, among other cues, observe the direction they point their legs and feet. They can show you if they are welcoming your attention, even if they are crossed. Notice the direction of this attractive woman's left leg and foot.

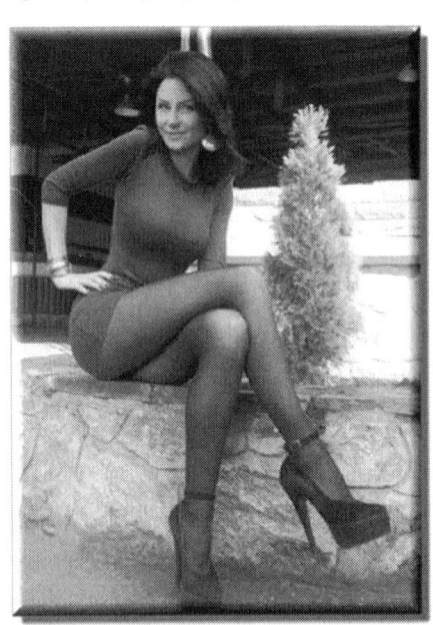

I said her left leg and foot...

HANDS

Showing your hands and keeping them in the open tends to create more trust. When our ancestors confronted each other for the first time, they never knew if the other was carrying a weapon. Therefore, to establish trust, they showed their hands as much as possible and kept them in the open.

To show even more trust, they exposed the palms of their hands. If a woman starts exposing her wrists to you, that's a great sign because it's telling you that she really trusts you and she is making herself vulnerable to you.

That's why it's so important to keep your hands and nails looking their best, because you can bet she is going to be inspecting them very closely. It's a huge indicator of your grooming habits, and besides, if your hands and nails are not clean and well groomed, the chances of you touching her or putting them on or in her are going to be very limited.

Your hands are another way of communicating non-verbally. For example, someone who sits with their hands on their lap is probably saying, "I am patient," or "I am listening," whereas hands on the hips could mean, "I'm getting impatient, let's move along."

Your hands may be used to your advantage by subconsciously compelling a woman to get closer to you. If you keep your hands in view or even keep the palms of your hands open and extended toward the woman, this has the effect of drawing her in closer to you.

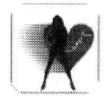

You can also use them to focus interest on her. For example, if you are sitting at a table you could clasp your hands together, and point them in her direction. You may also use your hands to gesticulate when telling a story or emphasizing a point. It will make you a more interesting and dramatic speaker.

If you're trying to show confidence and power, you can steeple your hands while resting your elbows on the chair arms or table. It also conveys wisdom, intelligence, or deep thought.

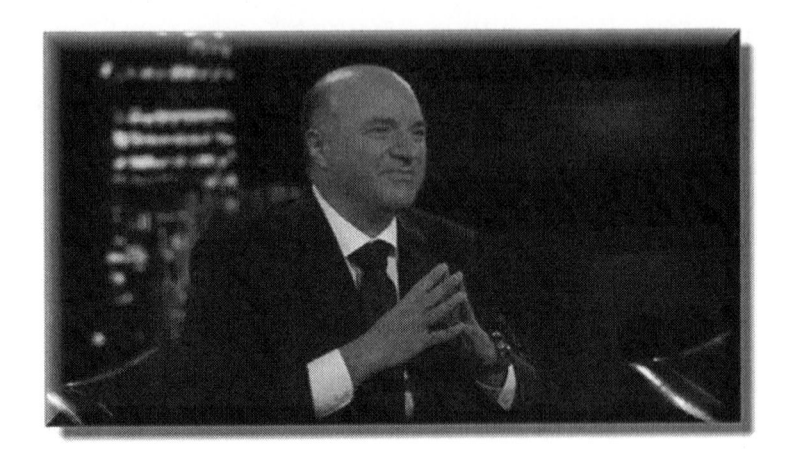

When you're standing or leaning, you can put your thumbs in your pockets or waistband and have your fingers point towards your genitals. This is a pose you may want to practice in the mirror so when you do it, you know you look cool and masculine.

5.2 PROXEMICS (THE USE OF SPACE)

Studies conducted at the University of Texas have shown that we tend to lean forward toward people we like and we move our entire body closer to theirs as well.

Haven't you ever noticed yourself making a slight detour across a supermarket aisle or changing lanes in traffic to get closer or to get a better look at some attractive woman? A self-confident man will not hesitate to get closer to a woman when talking to let her know that he is interested in her.

So, to develop a warm and pleasing personality, move your body physically closer to her, sit or stand next to her, but not so close as to crowd her. Be keenly aware of the spatial boundaries she's setting so you don't make her feel uncomfortable. According to Dr. Wassmer, most people who are shy will pull up or lean back when they don't want to be discovered or when they don't want to intrude on the space of another.

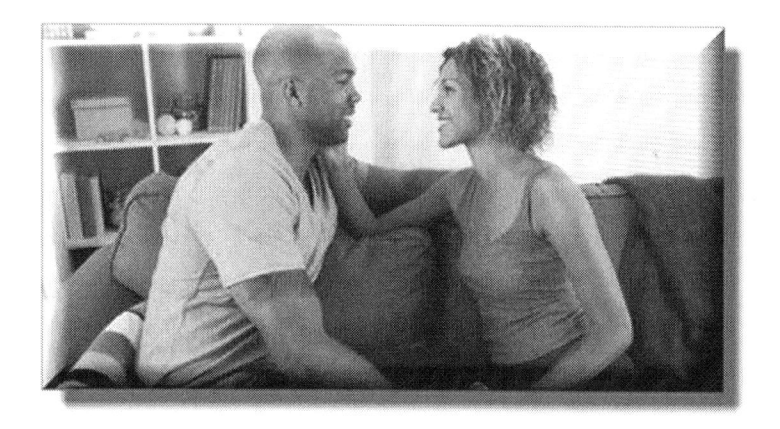

Other people, unfortunately, may interpret the backward lean as a sign of disapproval or disinterest. So if you want to show a woman you're interested in her, lean forward and nod when talking or listening to her. If you are standing, turn your head towards her. It lets her know that you want to know everything she is saying.

So as you can see, the whole mating and courting ritual is really a dance – it's a tease, where you show interest to draw her in, and then when she starts to back off slightly – you demonstrate disinterest that has the tendency to draw her back towards you. It's a primal, subconscious, tug of war mating ritual and it exists throughout the animal kingdom.

Women use the allure of sex to tease and draw in men, and they instinctively know how to use it to make you pursue them. You should use your body language and high status humor to do the same now that you know how to use it.

Women love for you to tease them; in fact, it's really a preamble to how you make love to a woman. The tease increases and intensifies desire. The best way to arouse sexual desire in a woman is playfully tease her in and out of the bedroom.

MOVE IN CLOSER

Ovid, a first century Roman poet whose two thousand year old book *Ars Amortoria* (The Art of Loving), knew back even then how to enhance one's appeal by inconspicuously moving in closer: (translated from Latin)

And if a speck of dust, as well it may, Drop on her lap, flick the speck away,

And if there's none, then flick what isn't there, seize any pretext for a show of care.

A great way to move in closer is to whisper in her ear. Whisper anything and it sounds sexy and intimate. It doesn't have to be anything profound or intellectual, something as simple as *"You might be attractive but I don't know if you're right for me."*

Alternatively, you might try something like, *"You know what they say about women who wear red lipstick,"* or you can even whisper, *"Are we having fun yet?"* You can try a number of things to get closer to her so you can exchange pheromones and make the transition to a kiss much easier.

Other ways you can get closer are:

1. Gently reach for her wrist so you can read her watch

2. Gently brush an eyelash from her face

3. Tell her how much you like her perfume, then move in close enough to smell it on her neck

4. Tell her how much you like her necklace or ring, then move in close enough to examine it

5. Gently brush her hair from her face or off her ear

6. Brush off the speck of lint that is or isn't there

WAYS TO MOVE HER CLOSER TO YOU:

7. Ask her to straighten your collar or tie if you have one

8. Ask her to see if there is something in your eye, and then steal a quick kiss on her cheek

9. Grab her hand and spin her around as if you're about to dance with her

10. Ask her to check out your contact lens – even if you aren't wearing any

TOUCHING

If you want to increase attraction and lay the groundwork for more intimacy – learn how to touch her in a non-threatening way.

Several studies have shown that touching is important to survival. Humans, rats, and many other types of animals can develop mental and physical disorders; some may even die without touch.

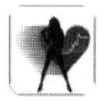

Touching is a vital part of our existence. There is no reason to feel inhibited about touching others. Touching is the most intimate of our five senses and we all need to touch and be touched. Touching coupled with eye contact is usually a good indicator of caring.

Touching is an extremely effective way to communicate non-verbally. The way you touch can also have a special meaning. One way to indicate companionship is to put your arm around her waist or shoulder. Holding her waist while you guide her into a car or into a door is an extremely powerful way to increase instant attraction.

You might even try placing your open hand on her knee when talking or listening to her. Gently caressing her shoulder or arm is a good way to show affection. So, when talking or listening to a woman, don't be afraid to reach out and touch her arm or gently place your hand on her knee for a few seconds. The more familiar you become with her, the more you should feel free to touch her.

If she likes you, I'm sure she won't mind. In fact, she will undoubtedly enjoy your touch and it may even slightly turn her on. You should make it a point to touch or lightly caress her at least once every time you see her, even if you don't say anything to her.

It is another way of telling her, "I like being with you and you make me feel good." Touching yourself is also a very powerful way to communicate non-verbal sex appeal.

MIRRORING AND MATCHING

Use your body to create a subtle and closer bond between you by adopting a similar posture. Psychiatrists, salespeople, and pickup artists commonly use this in order to create familiarity and trust with others.

For example, if she crosses her legs while sitting, you may do the same. If she leans against the wall, go ahead and lean against the wall too. Don't be too obvious.

There are three main things to try to match in order to be in synch and create trust and attraction with a woman:

1. Her posture and body movements

2. The rhythm and cadence of her speech

3. Using the same words she uses

You may subconsciously have already noticed yourself doing this to someone you've been attracted to. These types of subconscious signals we send out attract people to each another. Once you are in synch, you'll notice that you can even take the lead and she will start to model your behavior as well.

5.3 PARALANGUAGE (VOICE QUALITY OR DELIVERY)

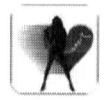

One of the most important elements of high status humor is your delivery whenever you're about to say something humorous. I've carefully studied the coolest and best high status comedians, and following are the most common traits they share:

1. Avoid broadcasting your intent. They disguise the punch line with a straight set up. Nothing ruins humor more than broadcasting your intent before you begin.

2. Minimize smiles and laughter - They don't smile much if ever and when they do, it's minimal. It has to be something hilarious and outrageous. Others should have to earn your approval, that way it becomes more valuable and they will try harder to get it.

3. Don't laugh at your own humor or punch lines – High status comedians especially don't laugh out loud at their own humor or punch lines.

4. Keep eye blinking rate to a minimum – it helps to escalate tension and attraction.

5. Make direct eye contact - When they are telling a humorous story or setting up a joke, they look directly at the person and make strong eye contact as if they are telling them a very serious and personal story.

6. Look away after the punch line - When they deliver the punch line, they look away or off in the distance, and if they have to laugh or smile, they do it in a way that says it's just for their amusement only, and not intended to make everyone else laugh.

If you examine humor, you'll find that what makes us laugh is the buildup of tension and the release. It's as if you take them down a road in one direction, and you suddenly end up somewhere absurd – or like walking a typical crony-capitalist politician onto a red carpet pretending to honor their work, then pulling the rug out from under them.

Now that's funny.

PRESELECTION

Preselection is the impression you make on a woman even before you meet her. In other words, even before you personally meet a woman, she is already analyzing you. Her opinion of you could be the result of your body language and your appearance, the way others treat you, and what she may have heard from others about you.

There are many ways to make a good impression prior to meeting someone, and one way is your reputation. In essence, your reputation is a first impression, and your reputation is likely to shape others' opinion of you even if it is not true.

We are primed to see a person as living up to his or her reputation, just as we are ready to laugh at a comedian even before he says something funny. For example, merely by looking at someone like Larry the Cable Guy or Chris Rock makes you want to crack up even before they open their mouth.

Of course, it is not always possible or very easy to prime the person you are trying to impress with all of your outstanding qualities, but in certain circumstances like a blind date or party, you can do it.

If you have the reputation of being a human alpha male that other women want, then that makes you desirable to other women because you have been "preselected" by others. In the forthcoming section on 12 habits of the human alpha male, you will see those traits that attract women at the subconscious and primal level.

For example, in the intro when I shifted the Latin Lady to make it look like she pinned me against the wall, this demonstrated to others watching that I had high value, and thus made me appear more desirable to the other women. Women desire men that other women want because they are preselected.

In my other books, I show how you can do this by using a friend or family member (wingman) or when creating an online profile – but that's a discussion for another day. Here you're going to learn how to make the best first impression possible.

CHAPTER 6 - HOW TO MASTER A SENSE OF HUMOR

HERE'S HOW TO DEVELOP IT AND WHERE TO GET IT

In this chapter, I'm going to share with you what social scientists say about pickup lines, which types are the most effective, and the best ways to deliver them. I'll also show you several ways to develop your own style of humor by giving you several examples.

You'll also learn where to find high status humor and how to blend it with your own personality so you can incorporate it easily into your own style. By the time you finish this chapter, I'm sure you'll be eager to start thinking of all the humorous things you've ever heard and personally experienced throughout your life so you can begin to use this system and translate them into humorous ways to attract and connect with women.

THE FACTS ABOUT PICKUP LINES

I've always been fascinated with pickup lines because it's how you generally introduce yourself and it's usually your first chance to make a good impression. I've been experimenting with them for several years to determine what works and what doesn't. I came across a study about pickup lines that meshes nicely with my experiences so I'd like to share it with you.

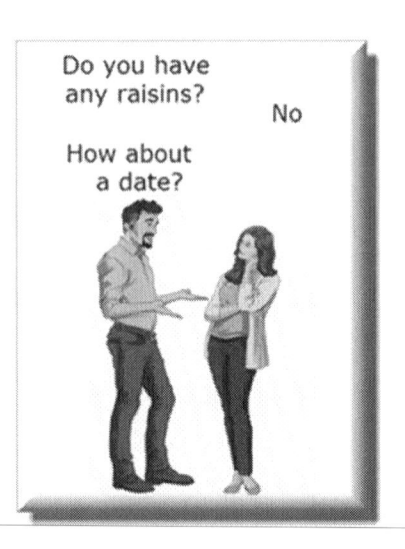

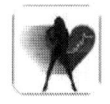

How to Attract Women With Humor

Social scientists in several settings and experiments have determined that there are three types of pickup or opening lines, and which types are the most effective with women:

1. **Cute/Flippant opening line** – These involve humor or kidding and generally require a high degree of confidence to pull off. You should typically use them only when you have first established welcoming eye contact, because you can crash and burn if you don't.

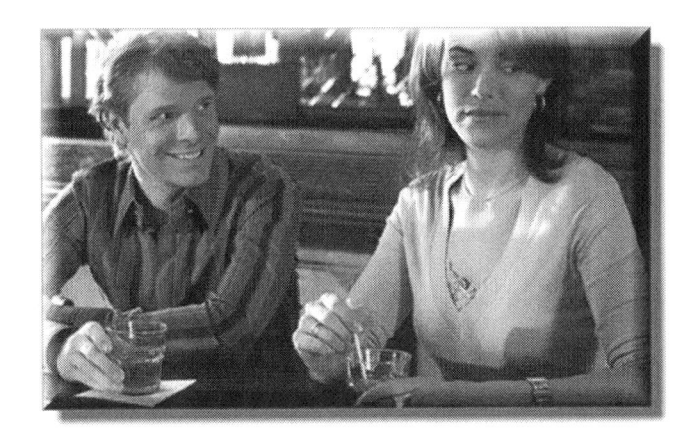

Example 1: "I don't usually let cute girls hit on me, but for you I'll make an exception"

Example 2: "I've been looking for a girl like you – not you, but a girl just like you"

101 | Page

2. Direct opening line – These consist of directly approaching a woman without any pretense whatsoever. The direct and innocuous opening lines have tested to be much more successful with women looking for long-term relationships. They are also easier to deliver, especially for the inexperienced.

Example 1: "Hi, my name is Buster Hymen, what's yours?" (Just kidding, I had to use that name somewhere; of course, you should use your own name if it's a direct opener. I could have just as well used Heywood Jablowme or Dick Gozinya – sorry I couldn't resist.)

Example 2: "Hi – do you mind if I sit next to you?"

3. Innocuous opening line – This is when you use something in your surroundings or you refer to something happening to start a conversation – for example:

Example 1: "Hi, would you happen to know what time it is?"

Example 2: "What's good to eat here?"

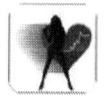

It's been demonstrated many times that women who are most interested in long term relationships respond best to direct and innocuous opening lines, while women who are interested in short term relationships or one night stands respond better to the cute/flippant opening line.

Studies have shown that in most cases, the cute/flippant opening line is not very successful. It's my opinion that most guys don't know how to successfully deliver cute/flippant lines, and that's why they tested poorly.

The studies also showed that when they were successful, they tended to work better with women who were not looking for a long-term relationship. Perhaps that is precisely why many men like to use the cute/flippant opening line because it saves them time if they're looking for just a one nighter.

The Cute/Flippant opening line runs the biggest risk of failure when the content is cheesy or corny, poorly delivered, welcoming eye contact has not established or used on women who are interested in a long-term relationship.

If you're going to use this type of opening, you should first establish welcoming eye contact and/or have supreme confidence when delivering them. Otherwise, it can be a recipe for disaster because it will sound to her deceptive and the person delivering it untrustworthy.

In my opinion, hybrid-opening lines for example cute/flippant/direct and cute/flippant/innocuous have the highest probability of success because they are humorous and direct or innocuous.

For instance, here is a cute/flippant/ and direct:

"Hi, do you know Leonardo?" She says no, and you say, "Hi, I'm Leonardo, what's your name?"

Alternatively, there is the cute/flippant and innocuous:

"Did you ever notice how it's always room temperature wherever you are?"

No matter which approach you use, you can be prepared to follow up with any number of generic humorous lines or cold reads you will find in the appendix of this book. With some experience and practice, you'll be able to blend them into the conversation effortlessly and eventually come up with several of your own.

Of course, other factors will determine your success or failure rate whenever you use any of these opening lines:

1. Personal timing of events – The positive and negative events surrounding her personal life can affect her mood and will thus likely determine your outcome. Even her menstrual cycle can be a factor. If she's ovulating and you have traits and characteristics that are desirable to her at an unconscious level – you're much more likely to successful.

However if you don't have the right combination of traits or characteristics, you may be rejected. Although she gets hornier during this time of the month, her heightened sensory perception due to ovulation causes her to become more careful to avoid men with traits she deems undesirable, and more attracted to those men who have them.

2. Personal blueprint of attraction – As we discussed in an earlier chapter, how much you appeal to her is determined on her personal blueprint of what she finds attractive. For example, the relationships she had with her father, ex-boyfriends, or even a movie star she just saw in a film or magazine will determine if you are desirable and whether or not your pickup line will work.

How to Attract Women With Humor

3. Your delivery - Your appearance, confidence, approach, and body language are all part of the unconscious formula she will use to determine whether she likes you and will want to engage you further.

You don't have control over her personal timing or blueprint; however, you do have control over your delivery. All of these factors combined will determine your ultimate level of success or failure. Your goal is to be as best prepared as possible and be aware of any hurdles you may encounter.

Finally, if you want to be successful with the cute/flippant approach, you need to be aware of these main points:

a. The content is good and not offensive

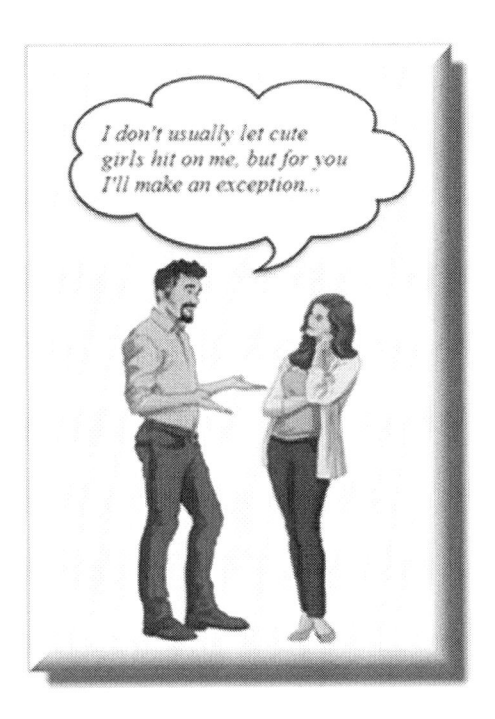

I don't usually let cute girls hit on me, but for you I'll make an exception...

b. You deliver it with confidence and the right timing

c. You've established welcoming eye contact and body language

There are unlimited ways you can create humor, but here are some of the ways I've found to be most effective and easiest to adopt.

HOW TO DEVELOP YOUR OWN STYLE OF HUMOR

THE PLAY ON WORDS

I'm sure you often experience times in a conversation when someone says something that may be interpreted in two different ways. Think of a way to respond to the unintended meaning, and do it in a way that sounds serious.

In this classic scene from Taxi where Reverend Jim takes his driver's test, you can see this technique used several times. His friends from work are there to help him. In case you don't know, Reverend Jim is a former intellectual who fried his brain from using too many drugs in the 60's.

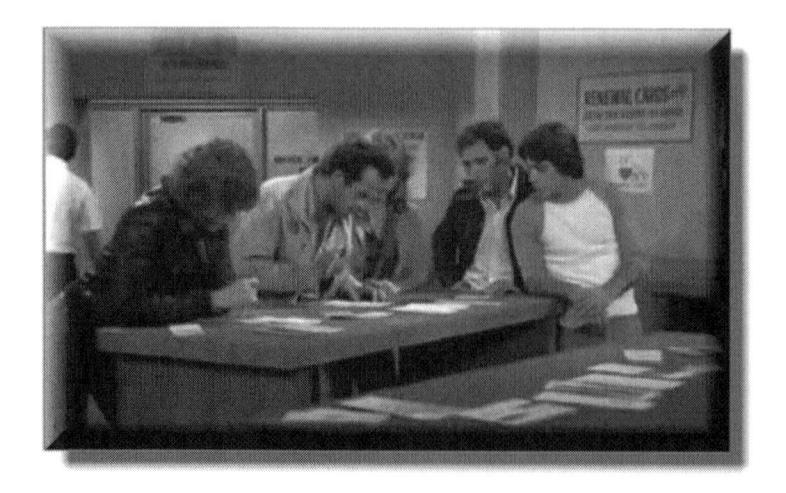

As he's filling out the application for his driver's license, he asks his friends to help...

Jim: Uh.... Eyes...

Elaine: No, don't put two

Jim: Uh....Weight... (Poised to write the answer, he accidently stabs his tongue with the pencil) Do they mean here or in outer space? Because there is a difference, you know...

Alex: I'm sure they mean here on earth

Jim: Whoo – this is the most reading I've done in years...

Bobby: Here, let me help you out. Have you ever experienced loss of consciousness, hallucinations, dizziness, convulsive disorders, fainting or periods of loss of memory?

Jim: Hasn't everyone?

Bobby: Mental Illness or narcotic addition?

Jim: That's a tough choice…

Elaine: Put no…

Bobby: OK, that's it – are you ready for the test?

Jim: What? I thought this was the test!

Elaine: No this is just the application!

Jim: Oh man!

Jim sits down to take the test. He is stuck on the first question and whispers to his friends for the answer.

Jim: Pssst – what does a yellow light mean?

Bobby whispers: Slow down.

Jim talks slowly: What…does…a… yellow…light…mean?

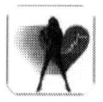

Bobby whispers louder: Slow down!

Jim shakes his head and talks even slower: OK – What……. does…….. a………. yellow………. light………. mean?

Bobby more emphatically: Slow Down!

Jim's exasperated throwing his hands up: Whaaaat………………… doeeeeees…………………. a…………… yellowwwwwwww

You have to see the scene to believe it. One of the funniest I've ever seen.

The play on words is my signature move and you can see it used in the intro. Start looking for instances in conversations where you can respond to or clarify a statement by taking the listener down the unintended path then pull the rug out from under them.

OBSERVATIONAL HUMOR

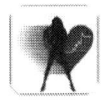

Observational humor is a form of humor based on the commonplace aspects of everyday life. Try looking for situations in everyday life that seem ironic or unusual. It's usually events based on the premise "Have you

ever noticed?" or "Did you ever notice?" This style can be highly effective because it allows you to tell a story, which is generally very easy to do.

In this classic standup routine, Jerry Seinfeld talks about what it's like in the waiting room of the doctor's office:

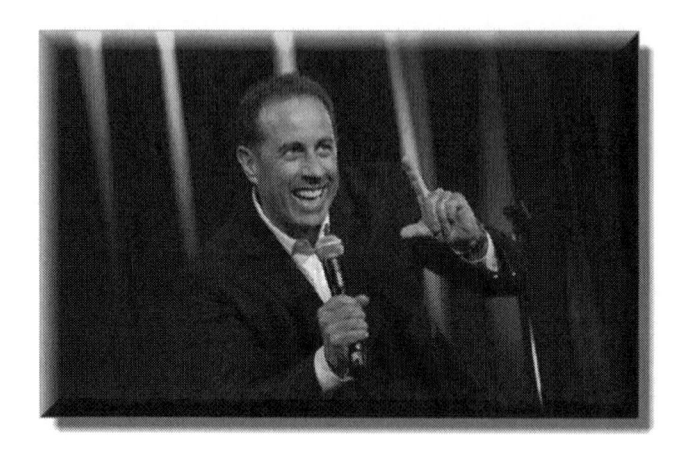

"Like when you go to see the doctor, you don't actually see the doctor first – you must wait in the waiting room. There's no chance of not waiting – that's the name of the room. You sit there pretending to read your little magazine but you're actually looking at the other people.

"I wonder what he's got." "That guy's a goner." Then you get very excited when they call you because you think you're going in to see the doctor. But you're not. Now you're going into the next smaller waiting room and now you don't even have your magazine!

"Get your pants off and get in there and I will tell you what I think" The doctor always wants your pants off. "Take your pants off. The doctor would like to see you without your pants." But I tell them I have a headache.

But I hate the extra wait, so maybe I'll start screwing around with some of his stuff. Maybe I'll turn that thing up a little bit, whatever the hell that does. I take all the tongue depressors out, lick them all, and put them all back in.

Yeah, two can play at this waiting game. Just once, I'd like to say to that doctor, "You know what, I'm not ready for you yet. Why don't you go back into your office and I'll be in there in a minute – and you get your pants off."

Pants beat no pants any day of the week...

Start looking for situations in your own life that you can make fun of. Think back on humorous situations that you can create a story out of, and try to use your own bent to look at it so you can start creating your own situational comedy. Start out with just a few sentences of a story and embellish.

UNLIMITED HUMOR ONLINE

I've been a fan of humor all my life and I try to watch and listen to as much comedy as possible. Science has proven that laughing can improve your immune system and help you to live longer. It can lower your blood pressure, reduce stress, improve your cardio health, boost t-cells, release endorphins, and give you a general sense of well being. Did I forget to mention attract women and make them want you?

It's no wonder that humor is a primal attractor factor embedded in our DNA. Look at all of the benefits it provides.

Throughout the years, I have accumulated a treasure trove of jokes, quotes, stories, and observations from albums, tapes, books, videos, and live performances. Today, it's so easy to find as much material as you want, and it's free.

As I mentioned previously, if you want to develop a better sense of humor, become more aware and start looking for it everywhere you go and in everything you do. Here are some great places to find unlimited amounts of humor.

    a. Watch your favorite comedians on YouTube

        i. Be alert to lines that you can use

        ii. Much of what I use is modified from other comedians

    b. Watch sitcoms on TV

        i. Whenever you hear a great line on a sitcom that you can use, write it down

ii. Watch sitcoms that match your individual style and personality

c. Do online searches for comedians alive or dead whose style matches your personality.

　　i. Personally, I like one liners, so I like to look up comedians like Rodney Dangerfield, Henny Youngman and Steven Wright

　　ii. Mark Twain and Groucho Marx have timeless and classic lines.

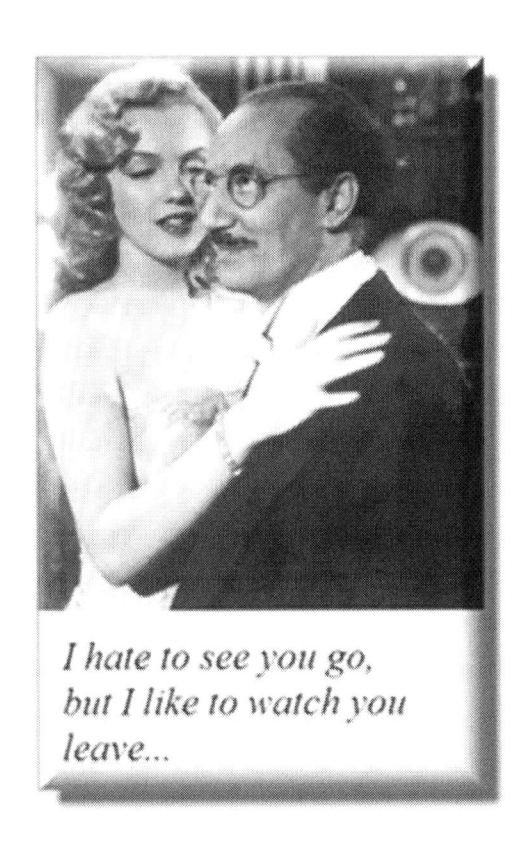

I hate to see you go, but I like to watch you leave...

d. Subscribe for free to http://www.newsmax.com/jokes/

   i. This website delivers to your e-mail box 5 days a week the best jokes from monologues of the previous night. It features late night comedians like Jimmy Fallon, Jimmy Kimmel, John Stewart, and others.

   ii. It's free, and it's an excellent source of unlimited, topical, fresh humor.

e. Subscribe for free to http://www.Pinterest.com

   i. Pinterest is an incredible place for humorous lines, pictures, and cartoons.

   ii. You can easily do a search for nearly any subject you can think of.

   iii. Search for jokes or humor on subjects she has an interest in so you can have a few pocket jokes and set them up in a conversation.

There's no excuse to run out of great humor when you have all of these great resources readily available. It's as if you have the best joke writers in the world writing great material for you to impress women and make them laugh.

Anytime you want to send a message, email or have something ready to say to a girl you're going to meet, go online and find a great joke or two you can use to make her laugh.

HUMOROUS STORY TELLING

Think about an event in your life that was hilarious or embarrassing. I'm sure you've told these types of stories to your friends and family many times. Telling a story is one of the easiest things you can do because you lived it. Of course, each time you retell it, you can embellish and add your personal twist of humor.

Following are few personal incidents that really happened to me. Each time I tell the story, the better they become because I improve the setup, I recreate the setting and characters more vividly, and my timing and punch line becomes more effective.

THE PATRICK DUFFY STORY

When I used to sell commercial real estate, I met with owners and gave presentations to acquire listings to sell their property. I recall the time I walked into one owner's office whose business I had been pursing for some time. He was on the phone. He signaled me in with his hand and asked me to take a seat until he finished.

Prior to a meeting, it was my custom to look around their office at pictures or mementos hanging on the wall to find a common interest. It's always best to establish a rapport first before discussing business.

As he was still on the phone, I noticed one picture on the wall that indicated he was into breeding horses for racing. I honed in on one picture that showed him standing in the winner's circle with one of his horses, and he had his arm around the famous movie star, Patrick Duffy.

When he got off the phone, I commented and asked him, "I've met Patrick Duffy before, so how do you know him?"

He replied, "That's not Patrick Duffy, that's my wife."

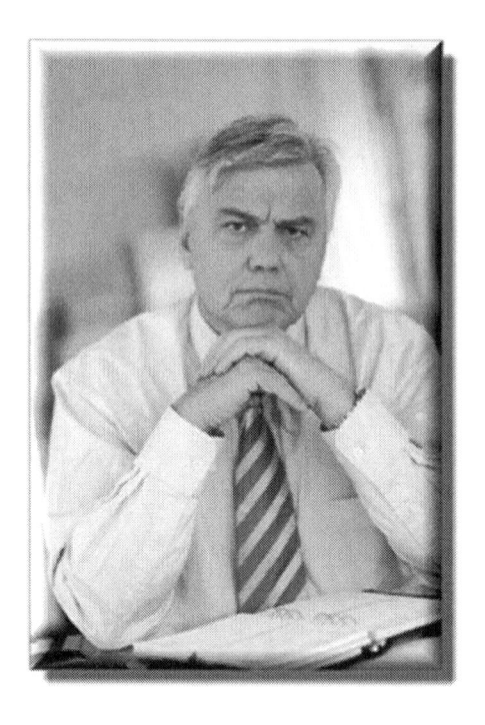

It was the longest most uncomfortable pause I ever experienced. The only reply that came to mind was, "How 'bout those Dodgers?"

I didn't get the listing...

THE INVESTOR

On Fridays after work, my friends in real estate would usually gather at TGIF's for drinks and appetizers to talk about women, sports, and tally up the weeks hits and misses. I was feeling pretty good after a few drinks when my cell phone rang. It was one of my most important clients, an elderly, straight laced, church going lady with lots of cash and property.

She called to tell me that she had to cancel our appointment the following day because she wasn't feeling well, and that she probably would be spending the weekend in bed. Having a sense of humor requires good timing, spontaneity and the creativity that sometimes only alcohol may or may not provide.

I saw my opening and without thinking it through, I replied instantly, "So you have to spend the weekend in bed? Is it going to be business or pleasure?"

She cleared her throat and ended the conversation with a long period of awkward silence.

Hey, I thought it was funny, or at least at the time it was... That one cost me a lot of money. One of the first rules of humor is to know your audience.

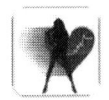

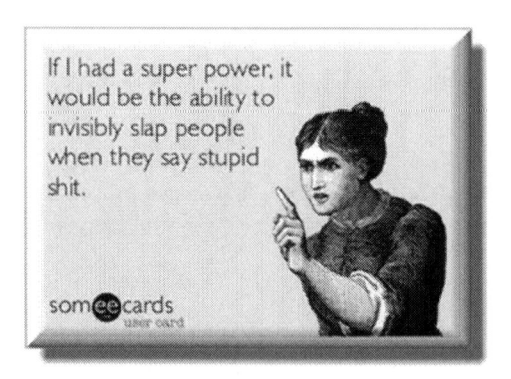

> If I had a super power, it would be the ability to invisibly slap people when they say stupid shit.
>
> someecards
> user card

"If I had a super power, it would be the ability to invisibly slap people when they say stupid shit!"

THE CAMPING TRIP

My friends and I invited a group of really hot women to go camping. It was getting dark, and after copious amounts of alcohol, my buddies and I started pairing up with our female counterparts. As I began to cozy up to my partner for the night, my eyes suddenly sprang open wide as I felt an aching churning in my stomach accompanied by gurgling sounds.

"Oh man," I groaned. Nature's distress signal sounded off like buzzers from a four-alarm fire drill prompting an instant call to action. It must have been those damn leftover fish tacos, and I knew I only had a limited amount of time to seek refuge in the nearest campground restroom, which unfortunately was about fifty yards away.

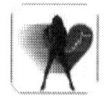

"I'll be back," I told my date with my best Arnold Schwarzenegger impression. It was a feeble attempt at masking the urgency, because even she had a look of concern on her face. I didn't even have a chance to put on my shoes. I ambled like a penguin as I hastily made my way towards the bathroom. The closer I got, the harder it was to hold in the unwelcome cargo I was desperate to unload.

It was dark, I was without shoes or a flashlight, and the closer I got to the bathroom; the faster my feet moved. I didn't see the large boulder directly in my path.

This is one of those stories with an open ending so to speak…

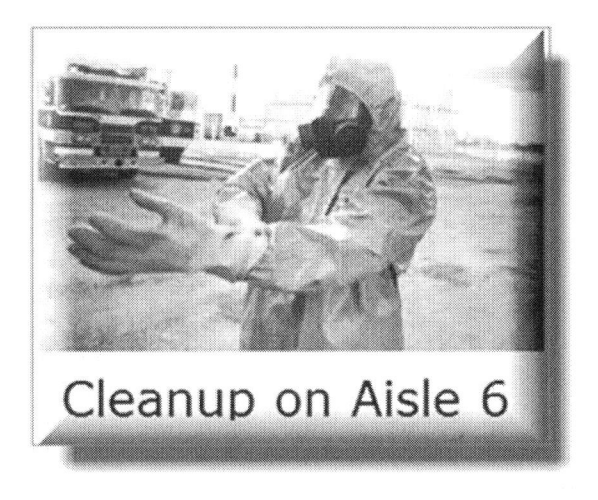

Cleanup on Aisle 6

Normally these types of stories you don't usually tell in mixed company, however if you can retell it with class and style, you can get away with it and come out smelling pretty good. Of course, timing is everything. This isn't the type of story you normally want to share on a first date, especially if food is involved.

I'm sure you can all think of embarrassing or funny stories that happened to you or others you know. The key to great story telling is the setup. A great way to setup your story is to ask the other person if they ever did something that has a similar theme to set up your story. For example in these cases, "Did you ever do something embarrassing or funny that caused you to lose business or a night of enchantment?"

Then after they tell their story, you say, "Let me tell you about the time I...."

FAKE STORY TELLING

I also have a repertoire of fake stories to keep your audience on their toes. A feature of great comics is to keep others guessing, and set up a punch line in a way those others can't tell if you're serious or about to set them up so you can pull the rug out.

Here are a few of my fake stories that you can use to lighten a mood that's declining.

THE BEER BOTTLE

You: "You won't believe what happened...I was partying recently in Vegas on the balcony of my 10th floor room and I set my beer bottle down on the rail. Some drunken guy stumbles and knocks it over the edge. It fell 10 stories and landed right on some poor guy's head and burst open!"

Your friend: "OMG -Wow – really - What happened to him?"

You: "Nothing, luckily it was only a lite beer!"

THE ACCIDENT

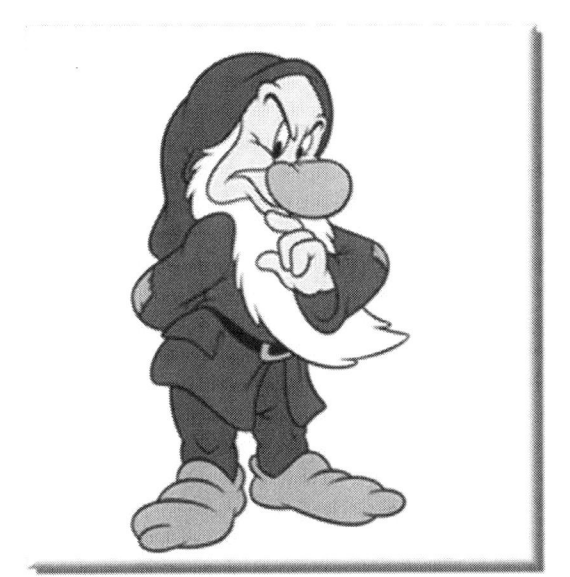

You: "On the way over here I got into a pretty bad accident. I rear ended this really little person – he must have been a dwarf."

Your friend will usually ask: "Are you OK? What happened to him?"

You: "I'm fine - I walked over to him and asked him if he was OK. He said 'Well I'm not happy!' So I asked him, "Which one are you then?"

STALL PHONE CALL

You: "I was doing and minding my own business in a public restroom stall recently when I heard the guy in the next one over say...

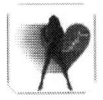

Guy in next stall: "So how are you?"

You: "I was at a loss for words, so I mumbled awkwardly 'er....fine....'"

Guy in next stall: "Are you busy?"

You: "uh, yes, as a matter of fact I am..."

Guy in next stall: "Do you want to come over?"

You: "uh – no – not really"

Guy in next stall: "Hold on just a minute honey – this weirdo in the next stall over keeps answering my questions...."

USE ANIMALS

One of the easiest and most natural ways I've been able to develop humor is to tell stories about my dogs as if they were people. I have a black lab/pit whose name is Coal, and his name in Spanish is Carbon – which sounds a lot like "Cabrón."

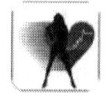

How to Attract Women With Humor

Cabrón is a name that most Mexicans use to call someone they're angry with, sometimes it's used with a sense of humor. The best translation would be jerk, ass, scoundrel, shithead etc. It has lots of versatility and the severity depends on the level of infraction.

When I'm around Spanish speaking people, I call him Cabrón and it's always good for a laugh. Coal doesn't seem to mind; in fact, he gives me a wink and a smile whenever others laugh at him. It's our inside joke.

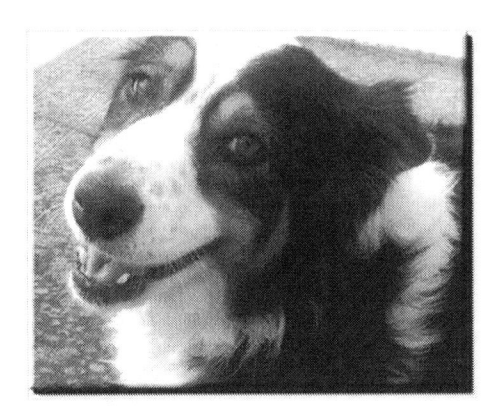

My other dog Máscara is an Australian Shepherd. Máscara in Spanish means more face, and it also means mascara – like the makeup women use to augment their eyelashes. When you see Máscara, you will understand why her name fits her perfectly.

I call them my security team because they are a two-stage alarm system. I live on a hilltop in a very rural area with a mile long dirt road. Máscara is the early warning system and stands guard outside scanning the horizon for any visitors. When anyone gets near, she barks to Coal in the house who relays the bark to me at my computer to alert me that someone is coming.

They also double as my personal trainers because every day just before sunset, they sit and stare at me until I take them for our daily hike. If I ignore them, Coal will nudge my elbow with his nose making it impossible to type – and he doesn't let me alone until I take them. That's when I call him Cabrón.

It's amazing how excited Máscara gets when I tell her we're going on a hike. She jumps up and down and runs in circles and back and forth

How to Attract Women With Humor

barking excitedly. Each time it's as if I'm taking them to Disneyland for the first time.

When I wake up every morning, the first thing I say to them is, "Whad up dawgs! What's on your agenda for today?" I swear Coal once barked in English, "Let's go to the doggie park, and check out the bitches."

They wait patiently by the bed waiting for me to impart my daily sermon of wisdom, and if I happen to repeat one I've said before, Coal will give me some attitude. He can get judgmental sometimes. We also have a deal where if I do the cooking, they clean the dishes.

Sometimes we'll even do Yoga together. Coal has a great downward dog, but his balancing postures suck.

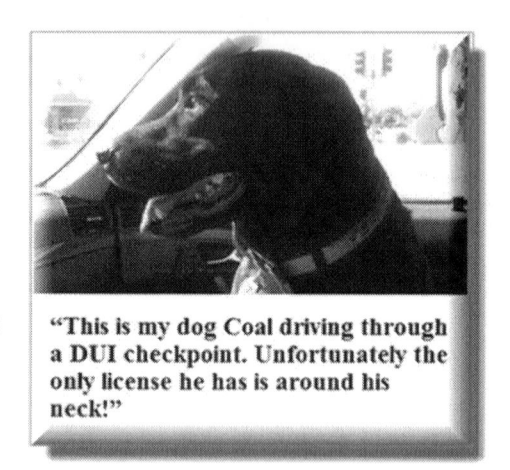

"This is my dog Coal driving through a DUI checkpoint. Unfortunately the only license he has is around his neck!"

IMPRESSIONS:

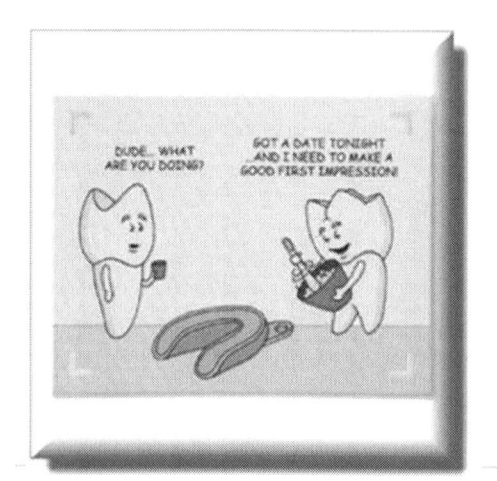

We have all done impressions of people we know, some of us can do them better than others. The only impressions I can do fairly well are at my dentist's office when they fit me for a crown. In the intro, I did a fairly good imitation of Mexican

Gangsters, and you have to admit it really adds to the story.

Some people have the ear to detect subtle nuances in others language and speech patterns. They also have the natural ability to imitate others, which is always great for a laugh and can be very entertaining. Just avoid doing it in a mean and spiteful way.

So if you're good at doing impressions, effectively try to work them into a story or to imitate playfully friends or family members, or in the work place, your boss. Just be careful to make sure he's not watching or a part of it. Remember the meme about people who say stupid shit, it could cost you.

COLD READS

A cold read is the process of making an assumption about someone based on an observation or opinion. Psychics make cold reads to gain a person's confidence and to let them know that they have a secret power because they know a lot about them.

Psychologists and Psychiatrists also use cold reads; and when used properly it can lead to a process called transference, where their patient becomes very dependent and attracted to them.

You can use cold reads to spark attraction or to get a conversation going with a woman or to even warm up a conversation when it starts to get cold.

Here's the formula:

1. You make an observation
2. You make a positive assumption. Try to make sure it's accurate or flattering.
3. Make a negative tease followed by; "But you know what they say about:"
4. Make a positive tease with your conclusion

Here are some examples:

The observation: That's a pretty red dress,

The assumption: You must get a lot of compliments on it

Negative tease: But you know what they say about women in red dresses;

Positive tease: They wear sexy underwear or none at all

Example:

"You have a cute smile; a lot of strangers must hit on you. But you know what they say about girls with cute smiles. They have great dentists, or their parents made them brush their teeth a lot"

Example

"You really look fit. You must work out a lot, probably yoga or kickboxing. But you know what they say about women who are really fit. They have a very high success rate. Or you could say, they are great in the....gym"

Example

"You seem intelligent. You must read a lot. But you know what they say about really smart women. They are usually attracted to guys just like me."

You can play with these cold reads to tease and challenge her in a flirtatious way. This technique escalates attraction and you can have a lot of fun with it. In the appendix, I have more examples.

In this chapter, we learned the facts about pickup lines and the best ways to use them. We also learned how to create your own style or brand of humor then to follow it with cold reads to spark more attraction and make a conversation more personal and interesting.

In the next chapter, you're going to learn the best ways to approach women.

CHAPTER 7 - HOW TO BE THE MASTER OF APPROACHING WOMEN

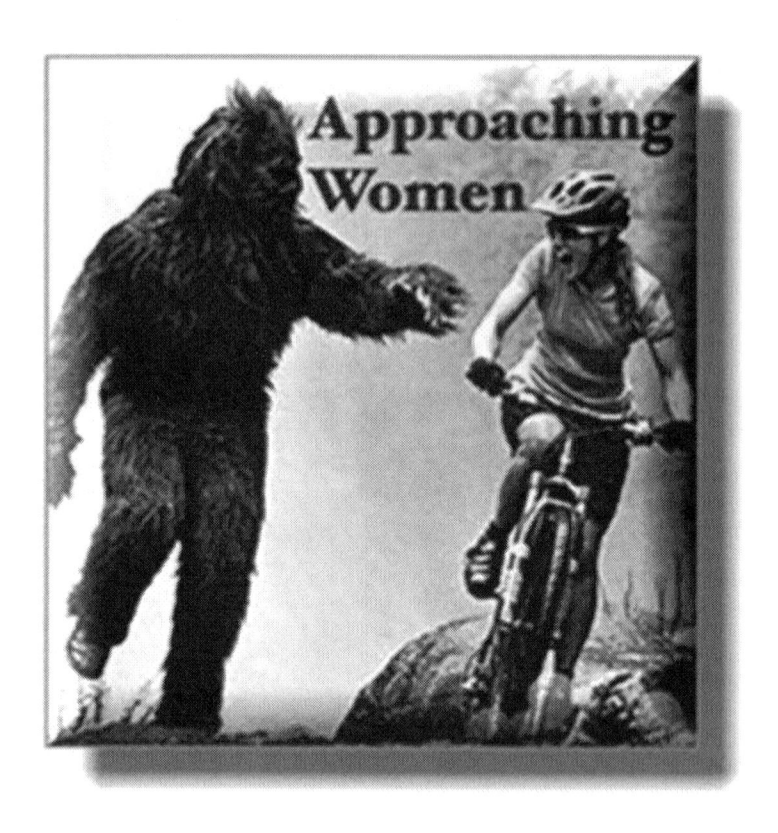

You've been given a lot of information so far, and now we're going to put it all together so you can approach any woman with supreme confidence, make her laugh, establish rapport and if she's available to date, walk away with her contact information.

When you have a simple, funny, and interesting presentation that you've developed, practiced, and perfected, you will absolutely become more confident and successful when you approach women.

I'm going to show you how to approach, open, then use high status humor as the ultimate icebreaker. A clever and humorous introduction instantly short-circuits her usual defense mechanisms and right away, you've made a good first impression.

You've immediately overcome that initial moment of awkwardness that usually accompanies meeting someone for the first time. Now it's much easier to establish rapport. When you start out with a non-threatening approach and add in high status humor, you can then say practically anything after that and get away with it.

When you first have the opportunity to meet or approach her with a direct or innocuous opener followed by humor that resonates, you've instantaneously created a positive emotion that you can build on. If done properly, you can establish immediate trust and likeability with the opportunity to take your connection to the next level. This all starts with a plan.

When you have a plan, it's much easier to smoothly transition from making contact with confidence and humor, then establish rapport so you can have coffee or a drink, then finally walk away with her contact information so you can take it to the next level.

You want to remember to close out on a high note with her e-mail address or phone number so she'll look forward to seeing you again. It takes all of the guesswork and anxiety out of it if you're prepared with a plan.

Once you've done it a few times, it will become as automatic and easy as learning to drive a stick shift that will drive you to the Promised Land. Of course, after you've done it a few times and become more confident, you'll be able to start improvising more and eventually you won't even need any prepared openers – you'll create your own.

However until you get to that level of confidence – you should have a basic, simple planned presentation or formula to work with. I'm sure you'll discover that when a particular approach becomes successful, it will become second nature without even having to think about it.

Wouldn't you feel more comfortable and confident if you had something funny and clever to say when the conversation stalled? It doesn't take much to ruin an otherwise stellar presentation then to have it awkwardly stall. Use a cold read like, "do you know what they say about….?"

Memorize a few funny lines and take it from there. With a little practice, each new line can start a whole new tease/challenge/humorous dialogue.

Some experienced pick up artists or experts might tell you that you don't need any planning or presentation because they forgot how difficult it was for the first few times. They already have the confidence and experience.

However, if you're new at this or want to try a simplified systematic approach that eliminates the guesswork and greatly enhances your confidence and success, then you'll want to practice and master the High Status or Affiliative Humor Beginner's Approach.

As you've discovered here so far, there are several ways to induce powerful emotions of attraction from a woman by using the Attractor Factors. Using strong masculine body language and exhibiting Alpha Male Behaviors are sure to draw and keep her attention.

Having something funny, clever or interesting to say in order to get it all started is the catalyst for making everything work together. It's the first impression and the straw that stirs the drink.

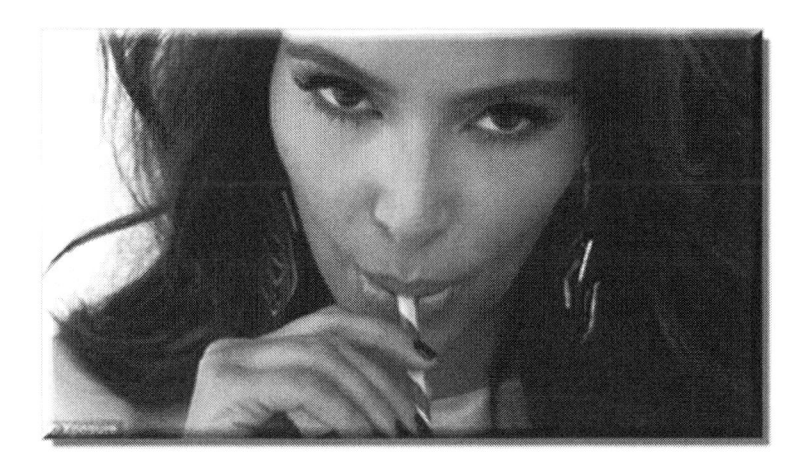

The ability to make a woman laugh can turn an average looking guy into one that all women want to be with regardless of your looks, income, or status. It tremendously compliments one's physical attractiveness. Knowing in advance that you have something funny to say greatly enhances your confidence and your willingness to approach women to make them laugh.

Quoting Dr. Arthur Wassmer in his book *Making Contact*, "All people are flattered and gratified by attention and interest. Rather than feeling that you are invading their privacy, the woman you address is more likely to feel, "How nice that you too feel I'm important." Contrary to your fear that she will think your question or approach is silly, their subconscious reaction will probably be, 'How intelligent you are to be curious about me."

In this next section, I'm going to give you a step-by-step method to give you the highest probability of a successful humorous introduction and minimize practically any risk of rejection.

THE HIGH STATUS HUMOR APPROACH

For the beginner, I've included the anatomy or blueprint of this simple formula to attract women with humor. I have dissected the approach to make it as easy as possible for you to examine in detail the purpose and expected outcome of each step. Remember – it's much easier when you have a plan.

You saw it demonstrated in the introduction, now here is the analysis and the play-by-play breakdown.

1. Determine your primary objective - Is it to get her contact info, invite her for coffee or a drink, just to flirt, or all three? Do you want to take her home? Do you want her as a girlfriend? It is a systematic process.

2. Gauge her level of interest - Does her body language tell you she is available and/or approachable?

3. Rehearse and visualize - In your mind plan your approach with a successful outcome.

4. Establish Eye Contact - Approach then stand or sit using confident masculine body language

5. Non-threatening approach – Be confident, but approach in a way that does not scare or intimidate her.

6. Use a direct or innocuous opener – or if you feel daring and cocky, choose one, two, or more of the many humorous opening lines you feel comfortable with and try to blend them with your direct or innocuous approach.

7. Play off her response –flirt, tease and challenge –use a cold read

8. Ask the right questions, setup one of your own humorous or fake stories

9. Build rapport - Ask the ultimate foolproof question to build rapport

10. Get contact # and leave - Get the e-mail address or number or set up the next meeting – leave on a high note

1. DETERMINE YOUR OBJECTIVE

Before you approach any woman, you always want to know in advance, what your purpose is. Typically, you want to get her phone number or e-mail address so you can contact her later and build the relationship. Do you want to just have fun by flirting and making her laugh, and maybe if you hit it off you'll ask for her number? Do you want to ask her to join you for a cup of coffee or drink with you at this moment?

You need to know in advance precisely, what your purpose is prior to your approach so you can consciously work towards that end. As Dr. Steven Covey said in his famous book "7 Habits of Highly Effective People," start with the end in mind. You'll have a hard time getting there if you don't know where you're going.

2. GAUGE HER LEVEL OF INTEREST

You really can reduce your percentage of rejection to zero and boost your confidence at the same time when you know that the woman you'd like to approach is going to be receptive. A new book claims that you can tell if she's interested in you by the way she moves her eyes.

Ali Campbell – Author of More Than Just Sex, says that if a man makes eye contact with a woman, she will often look away. But if you know what the glance means, you can tell if she would like to get to know you better or not. The reason is that *how* a woman looks away from you will tell you everything you need to know about the way she is feeling about you.

> *"If she avoids your gaze completely or if she stares directly at you with a blank expression – this is definitely not good. If she looks over your head with disinterest – this is also not good.*
>
> *If she looks to the side — to the left or right — this means the door is still open and a verdict*

hasn't been returned. She is searching her brain for an answer.

If she looks down in a way that seems to be sweeping the floor, this means that the lady is checking with her internal feelings. This is the one you are after. It's the holy grail of looks. It is a great indication that the female is interested in you. "

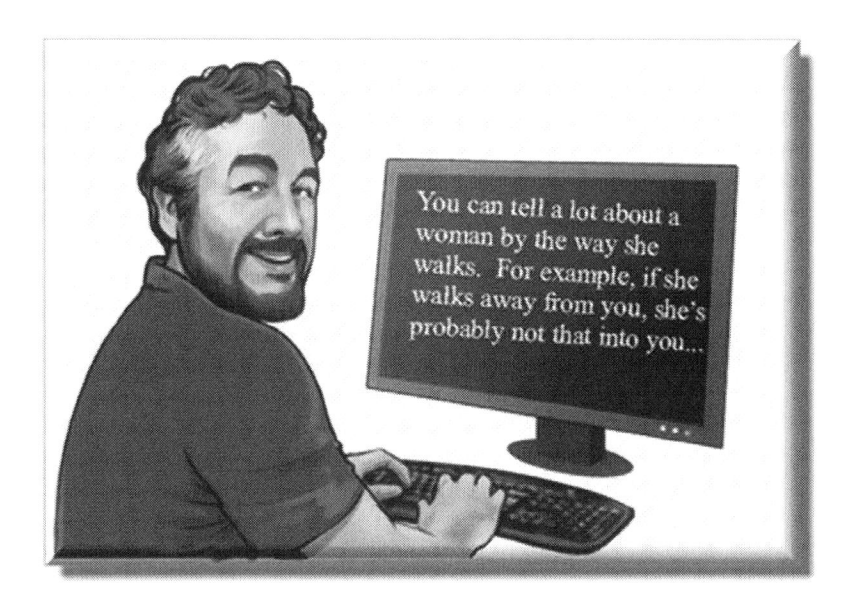

You can tell a lot about a woman by the way she walks. For example, if she walks away from you, she's probably not that into you...

In an earlier chapter, we also learned that women are generally responsible for starting conversations. We learned that:

- If she looks once and doesn't look back and doesn't smile — your chances may not be that good.

- If she looks once and smiles or blushes and acts coyly — your chances are pretty good

- If she looks twice — your chances are excellent.

- If she looks twice and smiles — you have a great opportunity in front of you.

With enough practice reading women's body language, you will generally get a good feel for how a woman is going to react when you approach her. In most cases, with enough practice and awareness you should be able to tell how receptive a woman will be simply by the way she looks at you.

3. VISUALIZE IN YOUR MIND A SUCCESSFUL ENCOUNTER

It's always a good idea to practice visualizing successful outcomes in your mind in any goal you want to achieve. Studies prove it will significantly increase the likelihood of you doing well. You want to rehearse in your mind walking over with confident masculine body language, using seductive eye contact, delivering your opening line like a seasoned comedian, her laughing, establishing a connection and rapport, and ending by you walking away at a high point in the conversation with her e-mail address or phone number.

I always like to give myself a pep talk first. To quote Mike Damone from Fast Times at Ridgemont High, "Wherever I am, that's the place to be." Now it's ShowTime!

4. APPROACH THEN STAND OR SIT USING CONFIDENT MASCULINE BODY LANGUAGE

When you're walking over to approach her, you want to make sure you're walking with relaxed masculine body language as we've discussed in previous chapters. You want to walk slowly, calmly, deliberately and with a purpose. Take long, comfortable strides.

Pretend you're delivering to her a thousand dollar prize that she just won. Don't try to disguise the fact that you're hitting on her. You want to imagine that she's already your friend and assume that she's going to be into you. You want to remember that you're doing this for your own entertainment, not hers.

5. ESTABLISH CONFIDENT EYE TO EYE CONTACT – STAND AT A 45 DEGREE ANGLE WHEN CHATTING

When you first look at her face, make solid eye contact and study her face a little, not too much. Stand and temporarily remain at a 45-degree angle to her so you don't appear too threatening or forceful. Show your hands, and smile very casually, and very little if at all. Release the tension from your jaw by relaxing it. Avoid any nervous behavior, like tapping your hands or feet and making quick movements.

You need to be aware of her body language. You also have to keep an eye out for when she's showing her shoulders to you. If she starts to face you with her hips, feet, and face – especially if she opens her hands and arms, and creates a direct, physical line of communication between her chest and yours – she is giving you very strong indications that she is interested in you.

When she starts facing you more, that means she is starting to trust and accept you. This is a good sign as it means she is opening up to you. At that point, you can start to open up to her more, but you want to remember to go with the ebb and flow. Give a little, take it away, give a little, and take it away.

If she starts twirling her hair, or preening in any way, that means she's starting to get interested in you. Other positive signs are mirroring and matching your movements, looking down at an angle and making more eye contact and communicating with you in a way that shuts everything and everyone else out – that means you're making very good progress.

6. USE ONE OR TWO OF THE OPENING LINES

Review any of the direct or innocuous opening lines in the appendix and pick out a few that you would feel comfortable using. (See the opening lines list below.) Of course, you can feel free to come up with your own. You should ultimately be the best judge of what works best with your personality.

Practice a few of your favorites and stick with them because you'll become more accustomed to playing off typical responses. Try to pick out ones that you can play with to have a spontaneous follow-up. Be aware of opportunities to play off her responses and try to turn your conversation into a fun and witty verbal sparring match that can really escalate attraction.

If you don't want to use a humorous or innocuous opener, you can always try the direct approach, "Hi, I'd like to meet you…" then follow it up with a cold read or question. If you don't want to try any opener at all, remember "Leonardo's Lead-in" – it's foolproof.

7. PLAY OFF HER RESPONSE – FLIRT, AND TEASE – THEN USE A FOLLOW-UP LINE

When you picked an opening line, try to determine which one will elicit a response that you'll be able to run with. Try to imagine how she will react to it, what she might say, and what you might say in return. Think of it as a mental chess game, or a verbal Jiu Jitsu match.

That's why it's good to stick to a few favorites because you'll get more practice and be better able to flirt, tease, or challenge them with your response. What's interesting about this approach is that some of the responses will become predictable, and you'll learn to be prepared with a witty comeback. Go back and forth and play with this banter until it subsides then use a cold read.

8. ASK THE RIGHT QUESTIONS, SETUP ONE OF YOUR OWN HUMOROUS OR FAKE STORIES

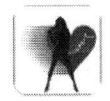

Listen very closely to what she says, because she will give you openings to play with. Once you've established the tone for flirting and you've opened up the possibilities of acting silly and flirtatious by first modeling this behavior yourself, she will be very likely to play along and say things that you'll be able to run with as well.

This type of flirting is a very powerful tool for attraction, as she will surely be having fun as well. You'll be amazed and even surprise yourself when you start coming up with spontaneous cute and funny responses. You can become very good at this with a little prompting from her once you connect. It will all seem to come so naturally. You'll be soon creating your own dialogue that romantic comedies are made from.

9. THE SIMPLE FOOLPROOF APPROACH

LEONARDO'S LEAD-IN

If you feel that you're not comfortable or confident yet with using any of the humorous opening lines I've suggested, then you should start off with the opening line that has never failed me. I'll repeat it here again:

> *"I picked you out of everyone because you seem like the perfect female to ask...I'm writing a book on love and attraction.*

Do you have a few moments, and would you be so kind as to give me your opinion on a few quick simple questions I have?"

Remember to sign up at the end for my free dating tips and a discount on my course on Leonardo's Lead-in when it becomes available. In that course I'll share with you the most powerful questions you can ask that will lead to lots of laughter and flirting, as well as questions that will cause her to become psychologically closer to you.

The book and course will be partially based on the famous controversial study that showed how two people can fall in love with each other by asking certain questions and performing suggested body language techniques.

In this chapter, we learned a step by step method to approach women with humor using the principles shown in this book. In the next chapter, we're going to learn the 12 habits of the human alpha male that will cause women to become attracted to you subconsciously at the primal level.

CHAPTER 8 - HOW TO BE THE MASTER BAITER OF WOMEN

HOW TO ATTRACT WOMEN AND MAKE THEM COME

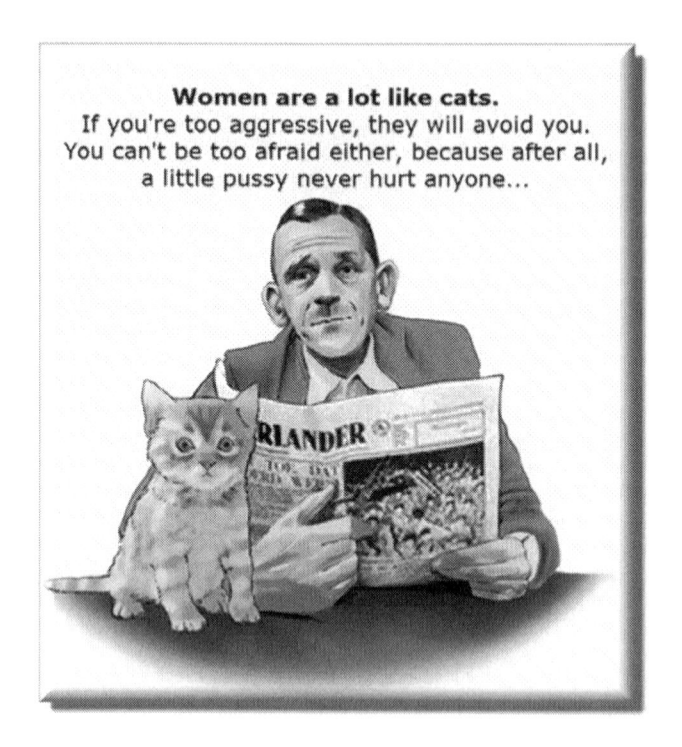

Women are a lot like cats.
If you're too aggressive, they will avoid you.
You can't be too afraid either, because after all,
a little pussy never hurt anyone...

Women are a lot like cats. If you're too aggressive, they will avoid you. You can't be too afraid either, because after all, a little pussy never hurt anyone.

In nearly all cases of the animal kingdom, the males draw females mostly because of strength, dominance, and adaptability to change, in that order. Because humans have evolved to use logic, language and modern social constructs; Human Alpha Males (or HAM's as I've aptly named them) thrive and dominate in modern societies by accumulating wealth, status and power.

Amongst humans, one no longer has to be the biggest and baddest to be desirable to women. The ability to develop resources and status has replaced dominance and strength as the primary attractor factors for women. Of course, resources and status are just the modern versions of strength and dominance.

A woman wants to be with a man who is fun, and one they can like and trust. They want a man who can protect and provide them with a comfortable life style, and be a good parent to their offspring.

The better a life you create for yourself, the more of higher quality women you will attract. Since the desire to have sex with beautiful women is most likely the strongest, instinctual force you possess, you should use that energy to motivate and inspire you to become the best you can be.

You can use your sex drive to develop resources, status, physical health and the confidence to attract women. As I mentioned in the beginning, our sex drive and intelligence is what made our ancestors (humans) the most dominant species in the world.

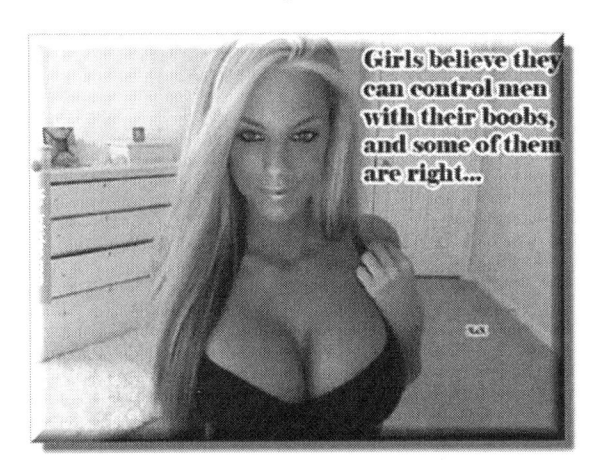

Women are hard wired – or genetically programmed to seek out males who have the fitness indicators I just mentioned. These ornaments are irresistible to women, just as women's ornaments like great tits, a tight ass, and a beautiful face are to you.

In addition, like anything in life – you can deliberately learn and develop these skills if you have the determination and desire. You don't need to look like The Rock or have the wealth of Donald Trump to achieve it.

What follows is probably the most important advice to attract women you'll ever find anywhere. It is what I strive for every day. Master these "attractor factor" habits and women will flock to you. Even if you don't currently have any of them, when women see you incorporating them into your life they will have the same effect still.

A high status alpha male uses "male cleavage" to attract women, just as a woman uses her cleavage to attract us. Listed below are the twelve most important Attractor Factors a modern Human Alpha Male can possess if he wants to attract women.

MALE CLEAVAGE

THE TWELVE HABITS OF THE HUMAN ALPHA MALE

1. The Human Alpha Male respects himself. He continuously strives to be the best he can be physically, spiritually, emotionally and financially. He prides himself on being confident, competent, capable, and clean.

2. He constantly feeds his mind positive, useful information that he uses to help others and contribute to society.

3. He sets very high standards for himself and others, and any praise he gives others is rare and they must earn it.

4. The Human Alpha Male respects others, and doesn't allow others to disrespect him. He treats everyone with respect. He stands up for what is right and always strives to do the right thing.

5. He surrounds himself with quality friends and business associates.

6. He avoids negative and disrespectful people and confronts them when necessary, but he never loses control of his emotions in any situation unless it's strategically necessary. He never says anything about anyone that he wouldn't say in his or her presence.

7. The Human Alpha Male has a commanding presence. He commands his body and posture to move like an Alpha Male, standing, sitting, walking, talking, relaxing etc.

8. He uses his voice like an Alpha Male by filling his lungs before speaking, pronouncing his words clearly and with conviction - and only swears or curses when appropriate or necessary.

9. He uses strong eye contact to convey confidence and certainty when communicating with others. He is kind, but not too nice – he smiles, but not very much.

10. The Human Alpha Male lives with passion and has a purpose. His purpose in life is most often his career. He is fun and interesting to be with.

11. He has a laser-like focus on what he's trying to accomplish and he makes it a priority.

12. He is passionate and extremely loyal to the important people and purposes in his life.

When you add in high status humor to the mix, it's like male cleavage on steroids, or female cleavage with a nip slip and/or a bald beaver.

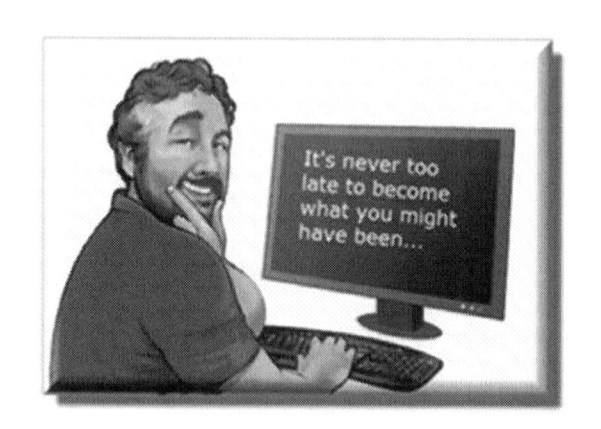

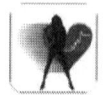

I guarantee that once you start practicing these behaviors and incorporating them into your life, not only will more women become attracted to you but anyone you come in contact will start treating you with more respect and admiration. Most of all, you will respect yourself more and your life will become more rewarding.

When you start carrying yourself with that air of confident masculinity, women will notice you more and give you unmistakable body language signals to let you know that they are interested in you, and when you approach them, you will more likely be welcomed.

We learned earlier that women are generally responsible for starting conversations by making eye contact first. The eye contact results from her approval of you, which basically is your body language and appearance.

GRADUAL APPROACH

Evolutionary psychology has taught us that the most successful way to approach living things we are interested in is in a slow, gradual, and non-threatening way. Whether it's prey to eat or a mate to meet, in almost every case we will have better success when the object of our desire feels that an encounter will be to their benefit and not to their detriment.

I recall an interesting story that perfectly illustrates this concept:

A herd of wild burros was creating havoc on nearby ranches and farms by destroying vegetation and eating feed meant for the farmers' livestock. The farmers offered a reward and the best cowboys in town tried to round up the jackasses without success.

Then one day a small, frail old man came into town in a beat up old pickup truck with a truckload of lumber and hay, which aroused the town folk's curiosity. They asked him what he was up to and he told them that he was going to catch the wild burros, take them home, and collect the reward.

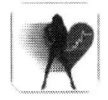

How to Attract Women With Humor

They all laughed at the old man because they knew even the best cowboys on the fastest horses and the best trappers with their newest traps were unable to capture the ornery critters.

About a month later, the old man came down from the hills with the herd of jackasses tied up and trailing behind the truck, and the folks in the town were astonished. "How did you do it?" they asked.

"Well, really 'twarn't nothin' to it," he drawled. "The first day I set a little hay in a clearing, and at first they didn't want to come. But one of the brave jackasses came and sniffed a little, ate some, then soon the rest of them came and ate the hay too.

"The second day, 'ah setted a post in the ground, put up a few boards and put some more hay in the same place. ' Shore 'nuff, them asses came back for more. Shore, they was kinda skeered at first, but they was hungry. I just kept addin' more boards as the days went by and' afore ya knew it, I built a fence around' em and they was mine."

If you want to attract women, make sure you use a mutually gradual approach.

When she rode her bike over the cobblestone street, she said,

"I'll never come this way again!"

Another way to demonstrate the mutually gradual approach is the twelve stages of courtship.

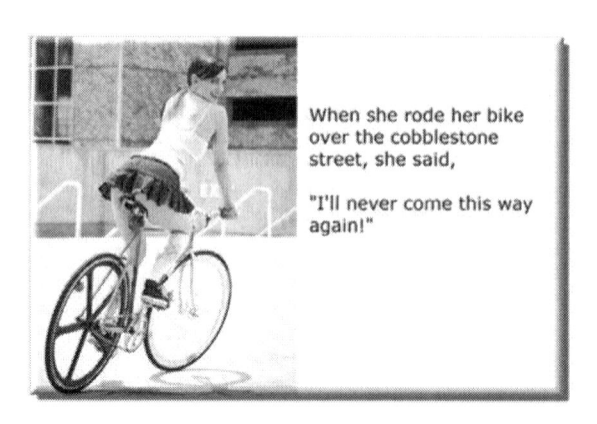

Dr. Desmond Morris, in his book *Intimate Behavior,* describes the 12 stages of human courtship:

1. Eye to body- We see people at a distance, and sum up their sex, size, shape, age, coloring, status, mood and quickly determine them as desirable or undesirable. If they seem interesting to us, we then move to the next phase.

2. Eye to eye - Strangers tend to alternate glances, because prolonged staring can be interpreted as an act of aggression and the other person may become angry or embarrassed. Friends tend to lock eyes, smile and greet verbally. If one or both strangers find the other attractive, he or she smiles while exchanging glances, and if there is a response returned, more contact that is intimate may ensue. A blank look in reply to a friendly smile will usually stop any further contact.

3. Voice to voice - Initial dialogue is usually small talk, and it gives both parties a chance to assess the other person not only through eye contact, but vocal as well. Dialect, accent, tone of voice, verbal thinking, and vocabulary give both people more information to decide if further involvement should continue.

4. Hand to hand - The first three phases can take seconds or months. Hand to hand can mean a simple handshake or holding hands for longer durations of time which usually means the relationship is growing.

5. Arm to shoulder - The first stage where bodies come into contact is side to side, which is the least intimate, and is the next smallest step to take that will be the least likely to be rebuffed.

6. Arm to waist - A further sign that the relationship is be- coming more intimate as the hand moves closer to the genital area of the female.

7. Mouth to mouth -This is a major step forward when combined with a full frontal embrace. There is a strong chance of physiological arousal at this point.

8. Hand to head - As an extension of the last stage, the hands come into play as they caress the partner's head, face, neck, and hair.

9. Hand to body- At this point, the male's hands usually begins to wander over various parts of the female anatomy and possible vice versa. Many females usually call a temporary halt at this phase if the bond of attachment has not reached a sufficient level of mutual trust.

10. Mouth to breast -This move is self-explanatory.

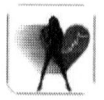

11. Hand to genital- As the hands continue to roam the body, the hands inevitably arrive at the genital region, where further stimulation takes place.

12. Genital to genital- The ultimate stage (for most people), and each stage will have served to tighten the bond of attachment a little more. According to Dr. Desmond Morris, "It could be said that we now perform the mating act, not so much to fertilize an egg as to fertilize a relationship." Of course, this isn't always true, but it makes a lot of sense.

In the following chapters, you're going to learn how to attract women to us psychologically, geographically and socially.

MERE EXPOSURE

A number of studies have shown that people and rats are more attracted to things they are familiar with. Repeated exposure alone is enough to enhance our attitude towards other things and other people. Social psychologist Dr. Robert Zajonc has conducted numerous experiments demonstrating the effects of "mere exposure."

We can use our own experiences to realize the effects of mere exposure. How often are you overwhelmed by a song the first time you hear it? Don't you like it more when you hear it a second, third and fourth time? How about the latest fashion in clothes or cars? Don't they seem more appealing to you when you see them a second, third and fourth time?

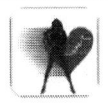

Well, the same principle applies to people. In most cases, we have to get to know someone before a close friendship can develop. Advertisements on the radio and television bombard us with their names in a favorable way and, you must admit, the more you hear it the more you begin to accept it and like it.

The advertisements sink into our minds subconsciously and we become more familiar with those names and brands. When it comes time to choose a product, we usually go for the ones we are most familiar with.

Love at first sight is a rare thing. I believe it is better described as "lust at first sight." Most loving relationships take time to develop and most people grow on us.

Sociologists Ernest Burgess and Paul Wallin conducted an experiment in the late 1940's in regard to "love at first sight." They learned that out of 224 engaged couples they interviewed, only eight percent of the men and five percent of the women recalled feeling a strong physical attraction for their partner within the first few days of meeting. Most likely, even fewer of these couples experienced "love at first sight."

The more she gets a chance to be and communicate with you, the more likely she will be attracted to you. You can accomplish this without having to say a word. Just the fact that she gets the chance to see you often will enhance her attitude toward you.

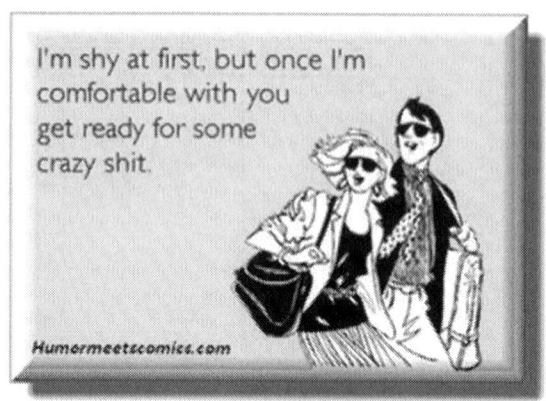

SOCIAL EXPOSURE

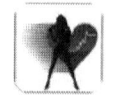

If you want women to notice you, you are going to have to make yourself more noticeable. In other words, make yourself visible. In my practice, I have met shy men who are extremely anxious to meet other women yet they don't want to make themselves more visible or available.

This goes for social engagements such as parties, weddings, nightclubs, dances or any other type of event where many people are gathered. You can usually spot the shy people. They are the ones who are off in the corner hiding under the dim lights. The shy people at parties will be reading, texting on their phones and hiding their faces behind them.

To become more popular you have to become more visible. Get out in the open where you can be seen. If you are at a nightclub, get a seat next to the dance floor or next to the main aisle where most of the people will pass. Seat yourself at the bar where most of the women order drinks.

Make yourself more visible by sitting in the areas of the club or party where you can get the most exposure. The same thing goes for parties; don't put yourself in an area of the room where nobody will see you.

Circulate around the room and try to gather in the places where you will become more visible. Make yourself more visible at any social event you may happen to attend.

If you're extremely shy and find it difficult placing yourself in the visible areas, start out in the less visible places and gradually move out into the areas where you are likely to get more exposure.

It is O.K. to start out in the less conspicuous places until you become more relaxed and more accustomed to the atmosphere, but it's not O.K. to remain there the rest of the night. You will not be likely to be discovered by hiding.

Strive to move into the areas of higher visibility. If you're at home complaining because you don't have a woman in your life, get out and get some exposure! In my opinion, the quickest, most economical and practical way to meet the most women possible in the shortest amount of time is through online dating.

In fact if you like this book, you should check out my course on internet dating, Meet A Mate Online. Internet Dating Reviews rated it the number one course on internet dating.

RESIDENTIAL PROXIMITY

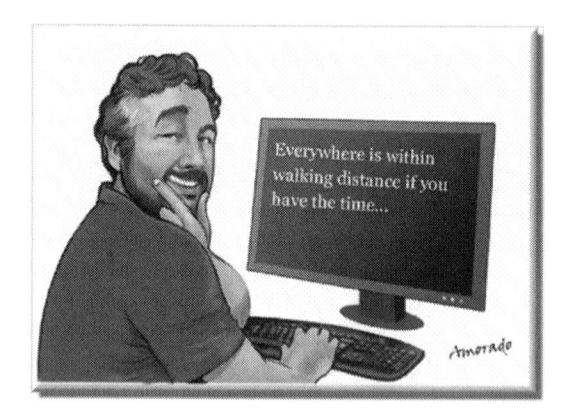

Everywhere is within walking distance if you have the time.

The architectural arrangement of the building you live in has an effect on your popularity. It can even determine who you are likely to become friends with and possibly marry.

For example, a study conducted at Massachusetts Institute of Technology by psychologist Leon Festinger learned that friendships and popularity could be determined by the design of the building and where one resides in that building.

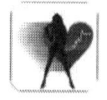

The people who lived near those places where people were more likely to pass by, such as the laundry room or mail box, were more popular than the people who lived in the corners of the complex who were not as likely to have frequent exposure with other residents of the building

Therefore, you can become more popular by living in a place where you get a lot of exposure. Another feature of the architectural arrangement in this study was that proximity mostly determined friendships.

In other words, friendships were more likely to occur between next-door neighbors than between people whose houses were separate from another house and even less likely between people whose houses were farther apart.

Thus, it appears that the distance you live from a person can make a great deal of difference in a relationship. The closer you live to a friend, the easier it is for her to get to your house, and the more likely you will be able to familiarize yourself with each other.

For example, if you live next door or even down the street, the chances of you running into her would be quite likely. The more you happen to run into each other, the more likely you are going to become friends. Familiarity breeds friendship.

In essence, the closer a person lives, the more value it adds to their appeal. You will have to think ahead of time, will it be worth it to ride clear across town (cost, time and hassle of traveling) to see Sally when I can go next door and see Susan?

A person has to decide the rewards he is going to get from the effort he puts out. If there is one friend who is nearby and another who is far away, the one far away will have to be more appealing or rewarding relatively to justify the relative cost of traveling.

Besides friendships, residential proximity also seems to determine whom we are most likely to marry. Sociologist A. C. Clarke interviewed 431 couples when they applied for marriage licenses. He learned that 37 percent of the couples were living within eight blocks of one another at the time of their first date, and 54 percent lived within 16 blocks of one another. As the distance between the residences increased, the number of marriages decreased.

The effects of "mere exposure" are obvious. We have to become familiar with things and people before we can really appreciate them.

At least part of the explanation for the principle of mere exposure seems to be the pervasive animal fear of the unknown. Although the unknown has its fascination as well, we remain unlikely to form positive attitudes toward unfamiliar objects until we explore them thoroughly.

It is through repeated exposure that familiarization takes place. We *gradually* learn that we can safely approach or deal with the object, and our initial confusion as to how to respond to it is *slowly* overcome.

In this chapter we learned how to strut out male cleavage, or the 12 habits of the human alpha male. We also learned how we can use exposure and proximity to make ourselves more desirable to women.

We are nearing the end, and in the next chapter, I'll be sharing with you my near death experience, and what I learned when my life flashed before me. You're going to discover the true purpose of your life and what will matter most in the end. You won't want to miss this.

CHAPTER 9 - THE REBIRTH OF MY LIFE AND CAREER

EPILOGUE: MY BRUSH WITH DEATH AND THE LESSONS I LEARNED
(Continued from chapter 3)

At the end of chapter 3, I promised I would update you to let you know how I got back into the business of coaching, writing, and showing others how to find love.

After my divorce, it didn't take long to readjust and pick up where I left off. Since then, I have had two incredibly sexy romances with fabulous women whose memories I will cherish for as long as I live, even though my life was almost cut short with a near death experience.

I mention this very profound and spiritual event because it gives me the opportunity to share with you what I remembered near the finish line when I started to watch my life flash before me. I want you to realize what the most important events of your life will be in the end.

I can personally confirm that it's true when they say your life flashes before you prior to dying. I was about as close as you can get. It's as if I watched a highlight film of my life so I could return to give you the answers to your final test:

What will be the purpose and meaning of your life?

Revealed to me were these answers and now I would like to pass them on to you like a cheat sheet so you can be prepared.

Your purpose is to become the best you can be so you can contribute and leave the world better than you found it.

The meaning is the joy and love you will share with family and friends, but most of all the passionate, sexual, and ecstatic love you enjoy with a romantic partner.

As I lay there near death, I remember the feeling of my spirit slipping away like a car battery slowly draining its energy. I then heard the crackling sound of an old movie starting as I began to see my early childhood flash before me on an old grainy black and white film taken with an eight-millimeter camera.

I saw events I had completely forgotten, like learning to ride a tricycle. I saw my mom bringing home my baby sister from the hospital, which means I was four years old at the time!

I must have been five when I watched myself playing in our old back yard pulling a wagon and wearing a Daniel Boone coonskin hat. I had a toy rifle strapped over my shoulder and I was secretly sharing an ice cream cone with my loveable dog and best friend Skippy. At the time, I thought I was in trouble for sharing my ice cream cone until I noticed my parents laughing.

The quality of my autobiographical film improved as I aged, continuing to show more of the monumental moments I lived.

I viewed the time I hit a home run in a playoff little league baseball game while everyone cheered. I saw myself laughing and enjoying dinner with our big family then arguing with my sisters afterwards over whose turn it was to do the dishes. I relived the time I maneuvered Kathy Lewis under the bleachers and kissing her for the first time.

I recalled the time I packed up to leave home and head off to Victor Valley Junior College. I relived the feeling of pride I felt the day in the locker room when the football team voted me co-captain. I experienced the thrill of victory when the referee raised my hand upon winning the 177-pound collegiate wrestling championship.

I saw me signing books and receiving applause at speaking events. I relived the times I gave dating advice and interviews on TV and radio – back before anyone else was doing it.

Even with the modest fame and fortune I received, I have to say the greatest sense of joy and happiness I experienced were highlights of the special times and love I shared with my children, family and closest friends. This reenactment of love and bonding with the closest people in my life overwhelmed me and literally brought me to tears. As I lay in the hospital bed fading in and out of consciousness, I was ready to go and it was OK.

I must also confess that distinctly apart from the happiness and joy from family and friends I experienced, the most physically pleasurable and monumental memories were incredible romances and sexual experiences I shared with the many beautiful women throughout my life.

While reliving all of these near death "This is your life" moments, it was surreal to experience the replay of a lifetime full of adventures while in reality only minutes passed. It made me realize how blessed I have been to experience so many of life's greatest gifts.

What is even more amazing is how unafraid I was to die and my only regret at the time was I didn't want my family and friends to be sad because up until that point, I lived such a great life.

Had I not developed the skills I'm sharing here, I truly feel my life would be diminished by at least a third. Much of my best times were of the special relationships and encounters I experienced with the incredible women in my life.

As I lay there near death, I'm swearing to you that I began to hear Julio Iglesias and Willie Nelson start singing to me, "To all the Girls I've Loved Before" as if it was my swan song.

I remember thinking, "I just hope the fat lady isn't on deck warming up!"

In case you haven't yet noticed, I miraculously survived. This experience and realization gave me the motivation to share with you what I have learned because I would hate to see you miss the most important parts of your life.

I'm talking about the pleasure of having intense, romantic, physical, loving relationships with sexy, beautiful women who adore you and ones that you can truly adore and appreciate as well.

My vision and desire is that this information will cause you to achieve some of your wildest unfulfilled fantasies with women and ultimately find the woman of your dreams and fulfill the purpose of your life. Maybe then, you'll be able to pass on to your next destination with a smile on your face recalling your own highlight film.

It's never too late to embellish your obituary....

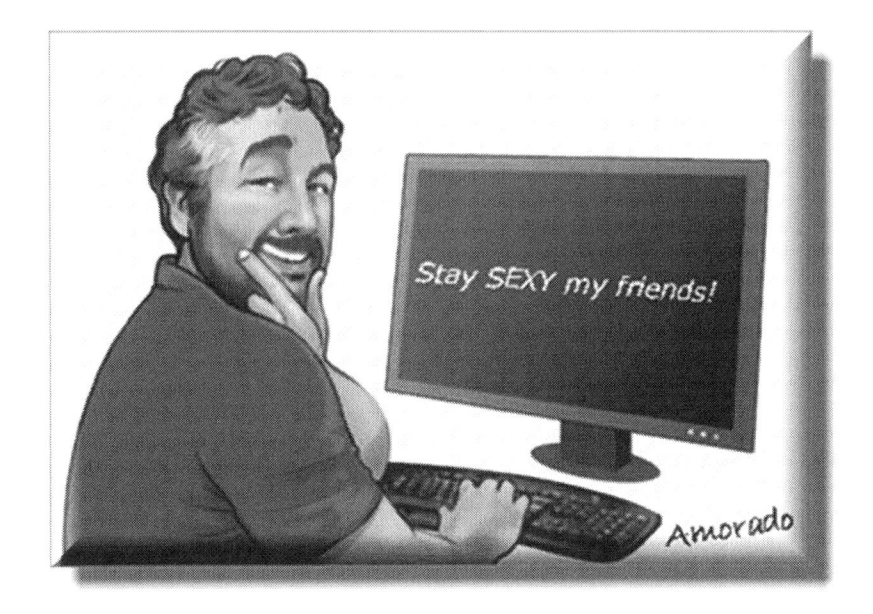

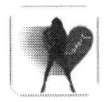

If you liked this book, I would greatly appreciate a review on my Amazon page. You can reach it here:

The link to my Amazon.com Review page is:
Bit.ly/HowToAttractWomenReview

I want to thank you for having the faith in me to let me help you. I've also set some time aside to help you out personally.

What problems have you been experiencing with meeting, attracting or approaching women? I've been there myself and I wish I had someone who could give me free personal advice. That's my offer for you and there's no catch for this. Simple pure free advice for you. And if you feel I've wasted your time I'll send you a check of $200.

Either way, you come out ahead. This offer will expire at midnight, December 31st, 2015, and I'll reevaluate it at that time depending on my availability.

Drop me an e-mail here Leonardo@TheCompanionator.com and I'll get back to you ASAP.

But wait, there's still more!

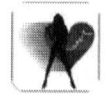

A brief note to let you know that the audio book version is unabridged, meaning that in order for me to produce it, it has to follow word for word what is in this book version. So if you're listening, the remaining part of this chapter is a breakdown of my other books, courses, videos and software if you'd like to know more about me.

You can access it all by going to www.TheCompanionator.com

Following this final chapter is the appendix where I've listed some of my favorite lines to open, keep conversations going, and escalate your date to the bedroom. Note that some may work for you, others may not depending on your personality and the setting.

Leonardo "The Companionator" Bustos programs, books, coaching and dating software helps you meet and fall in love with your ultimate love match

---

THE COMPANIONATOR WEBSITE

www.TheCompanionator.com

Sign up here for your free sneak peek at the upcoming "Leonardo's Lead-in" course that teaches you the ultimate pickup line guaranteed to help you approach any woman, anytime and anyplace so you can engage her in a humorous fun dialogue.

MEET A MATE ONLINE

www.MeetAMateOnline.com

Watch this video preview of Leonardo's # 1 rated internet-dating course online. This audio/video course includes dating software, e-book, and workbook showing you how to master internet dating easily so you can meet your best love match in the least amount of time.

LOVE ATTRACTION ACADEMY

www.LoveAttractionAcademy.com

Leonardo's upcoming academy is destined to be the Expedia of online dating. It is a hub for all of the best dating courses, books, programs and coaching that the internet has to offer.

MATE ATTRACTION PROGRAM SOFTWARE

Dating software to help you:

- Assess your dating strength and weaknesses in the <u>Self Assessment Questionnaire</u>
-

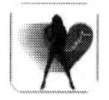

- Discover your dating desirability factor in the Self Evaluator Calculator

- Narrowly define your perfect partner in the Create A Mate Matrix

- Rate your dates in the Date Rater Evaluator

- Determine the best dating websites to market yourself in the Dating Website Analyzer

In the final chapter, you'll find the appendix where I've listed some of my best openers, conversation starters, and lines to escalate to the bedroom with humor, followed by my acknowledgements.

CHAPTER 10. APPENDIX

Below I have listed at least a hundred lines you can use to create humor. Pick a few that you feel comfortable with, and save them for opportune, random moments. Try to think of ways to fit them into conversations and eventually they will come to you automatically.

DIRECT OPENERS

Direct Openers

A direct opener is most effective with women who are more "conservative" and are typically looking for longer-term relationships. It is probably the easiest to use and doesn't require much creativity. You can always follow it up with cold read humor however a direct or innocuous opener is the type preferred by most women.

1. Hi, my name is .... What's yours?
2. I don't usually do this, but I couldn't resist coming over and introducing myself
3. Is anyone sitting here – mind if I join you?
4. I couldn't help but notice that .... You're wearing, and it caught my attention so I just had to meet you – my name is.....................what's yours?
5. "Excuse me, would you like some company?"
6. Aren't you on Match.com?

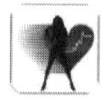

INNOCUOUS OPENERS

Innocuous openers

Innocuous openers are very easy to start with. Just look around for something to comment on and ask her opinion. Give her a compliment on something she's wearing. Caution - Do not make a comment on any of her physical characteristics. Studies have shown that is not very effective.

After opening with a direct or innocuous opener, be prepared to follow it up with something humorous. I've prepared a number of funny or silly things you can use – pick a few that fit your personality, and try to set it up so there's a smooth transition and not just some random comment.

1. At a restaurant - What's good on the menu here?
2. At a coffee shop – What type of coffee do you think is best?
3. At a bar – What time does the band start?
4. At a market – I forgot my recipe for Ceviche – do you know what I need or how to make it?
5. Standing in line – I'm going to be late for my meeting with the President
6. Walking down the street – Excuse me, do you know what time it is?

If she asks you, "do you know what time it is?" look at your watch, say yes and then walk away – of course, after a few steps you can turn around, give her a silly grin, and start talking to her.

You can ask her for directions – "Excuse me, do you know how to get to 3rd street?"

If she asks you if you know how to get to any location, you can say yes, then turn around and walk away. But of course, you will turn back with a sly grin.

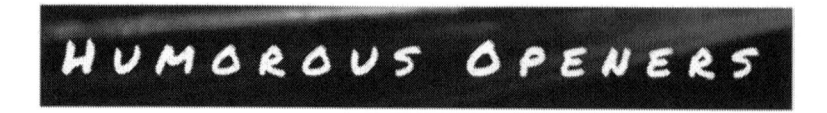

HUMOROUS OPENERS

Humorous Openers

Remember – Confidence and preselection
is the key to delivering any of these lines

Hi there:

1. Is your name Gwendolyn? (She says no, you say) "Thank god, I would never date anyone named that – my name is (insert your name).

2. Do you know (insert your name) by any chance? (And of course, she says no). You say, Hi, I am (insert your name), what is yours?

3. (Sit down with a deep serious sigh) "We need to talk....." (Then just look at her seriously and wait for her to laugh – don't worry – she will if you can hold a straight face long enough)

4. You remind me a lot of my friend Linda – but you probably get that a lot....I don't see her anymore, but that's not your fault.

How to Attract Women With Humor

5. I saw you checking me out – so – do you want to buy me a drink?

6. I saw you weren't noticing me so I thought I'd come over and introduce myself.

7. Don't look now, but my friend over there just bet me $20 I couldn't get you to give me three things.

Of course, she will ask – "What things? " You say, "Your e-mail address, a hug and a peck on the cheek. I tell you what – if you work with me here, I'll use the 20 bucks to buy you (lunch, drinks, coffee or dinner."

8. I can tell you're just dying to ask me my opinion about (pick out something in the room, then give an outrageously absurd origin or explanation of it.)

9. I don't normally let strange (or if she's really hot and you're in a cocky mood, say "average") girls hit on me, but for you I'll make an exception…

10. I heard you were looking for me. (Who are you?) I'm Mr. Right.

11. Did you come all the way over here to hit on me?

12. At my age (or "I've been really forgetful lately") I have to ask you, do I come here often?

13. I have to ask you, what's a guy like me doing in a place like this?

14. I was standing over there thinking about coming over here to meet you, but then I thought, what if we started talking, then you started to like me and then you got all hung up on me…..

Or the cocky funny approach:

15. I originally came over here to meet you because I thought you were interesting, but once I noticed that (pick out an article of clothing or

something about her you can tease her) you were wearing (or whatever it is you can tease her about) I sort of changed my mind. I tell you what – if you promise not to wear it on a date, I might get interested again…

16. I can't always talk to every woman that winks at me, but for you I'll make an exception.

17. Don't usually give my phone number out to just any woman, but for you I'll make an exception.

18. I'm writing an unauthorized autobiography – would you like to be in it?

19. I've got all the page numbers done; I'm up to page 246. I'll let you help me write it…

20. If I look familiar, maybe you've seen me at the movies. Just about every other week I watch a matinee at the local theater.

21. Didn't we go to different schools together?

22. Have you ever noticed how it's room temperature wherever you are?

23. Have you ever noticed that we get some type of weather out here every day?

24. Isn't it a nice night for an evening?

25. You look familiar, you sort of remind me of my future ex…

26. Have you ever had your palm read? (Take hold of her hand, and then mark her palm with a red pen)

27. Can you tell what material this is (let her rub some of it) its boyfriend material.

28. I've been looking for a girl like you – not you, but a girl just like you

29. (If she's smiling at you, walk over to her and say,) so, who's your friend? (You better let her know you were kidding – then make your move on her)

30. Nice shoes – I have a pair just like them

31. Can I ask you a quick question? Do you know when the attractive ladies are going to get here?

32. (Whistle at a girl near the one you want to get the attention of, then when she looks over, say) "Not you, her!" (When she starts laughing or is embarrassed – then make your move)

33. To a group of girls make a suspicious face and ask, "Are you girls talking about me?" When they say no, you smile and say "Why not?"

34. To a Girl who is alone, ask, "Hey, are you confident enough to accept a sincere compliment?" When she says yes, you say, "Good. So am I, you go first."

35. If you see, a really hot woman all dressed up: "I suspect that you're here not to see everyone, but for everyone to see you "

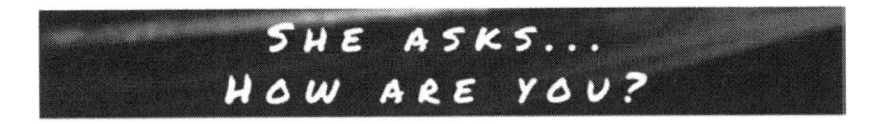

SHE ASKS... HOW ARE YOU?

She Asks... How are you?

1. I had a long accident at the mall today – I fell down an up escalator.

2. I've been reading a book about the history of glue – I couldn't put it down.

3. I went down to the store today and bought some used paint

4. I bought some powdered water, but I don't know what to add

5. You know that feeling you get the moment you lean back in a chair and you're about to fall over? That's how I've been feeling all the time lately.

6. I'm trying not to brag about how humble I am.

7. I can't wait until tomorrow. Why? Everyone keeps telling me I get better looking every day.

8. You say "I saw updock today" – she'll say, "What's updock"? You say not much Bugs

9. You say – "I saw a henweigh today – she says "what's a henweigh" you say about two and a half pounds.

10. You say - "I saw a dickfer today," she says "what's a dickfer" you say "Don't tell me you're still a virgin?"

11. I got a new dog today, and I named him stay – He goes nuts when I keep calling him – I say "Come here, Stay, Stay, come here!"

12. I got a new dog today, and I named him Ralph – so all of the other dogs can call him too – they say "Ralph! Ralph!

13. People are amazed that I have a talking dog that does Yoga – but he's not all that – his downward dog sucks and sometimes he lies.

14. I ask him what's on top of the house – he says "Roof" – I ask him what does sandpaper feel like – he says "rough." I then ask him "what's the skin of a tree called?"

15. I bought some batteries but they weren't included, so I had to go buy some more

16. I've been on a Tequila diet – I've lost 3 days already

17. Have you ever seen a full-scale map of the U.S.?

18. I don't like country music, but I don't mean to denigrate those who do. And if you like country music, denigrate means 'put down'

19. If I agreed with you we'd both be wrong.

20. "Nothing sucks more than that moment during an argument when you realize you're wrong"

21. Having sex is like playing bridge. If you don't have a good partner, you'd better have a good hand

22. When it comes to sex, I hold my own

23. I hate to see you go but I like to watch you leave

24. I always take life with a grain of salt …plus a slice of lemon …and a shot of tequila.

25. I used to be indecisive. Now I'm not sure.

26. They say you shouldn't kick someone when they're down – but that's the best time because they're closer to your foot

27. I sat down to have a talk about sex with my kid and I learned a lot

28. I have a lot of growing up to do. I realized that the other day inside my fort

30. At what age do you think it is appropriate to tell a highway it's adopted?

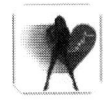

31. I dream of moving to India or Pakistan someday and becoming a cabdriver.

32. I dream of moving to Saudi Arabia to open a gas station.

32. I dream of moving to India and opening a call center for Americans.

33. I dream of moving to Mexico to sell tacos

34. I dream of moving to Viet Nam to open a nail salon

34. Relationships are a lot like algebra. Have you ever looked at your X and wondered Y?

35. I knew a guy who broke his nose in three places – I told him I'd stay out of those places if I were him.

36. I was so poor growing up that if I wasn't a boy, I wouldn't have had anything to play with

37. When I went to college, my dorm was so small I broke a window putting in the key.

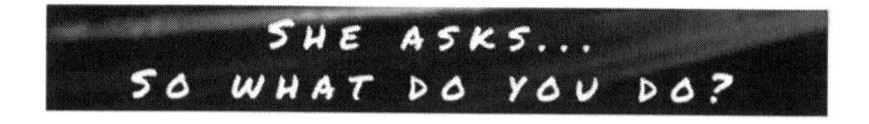

SHE ASKS... SO WHAT DO YOU DO?

She Asks...So, what do you do?

1. I teach sign language to the blind. I sign in cursive...

2. I work on an ant farm

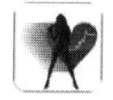

3. I own a chain of discount massage parlors – they are self-service.

4. I sell used paint

5. I work at a fire hydrant factory but you can never park anywhere near the place.

6. I'm a tour guide for a company that uses full-scale maps of the U.S.

7. I collect seashells – I have them scattered on beaches all over the world

8. I write phone books – can I have your number?

9. I manage a call center for customers from India

10. I write for Wikipedia – my ex got me started when she would always ask, "What's that supposed to mean"?

11. I box for a living – over at the supermarket

12. I'm a rapper – I work mostly during the gift-giving season

13. I edit for skywriters

14. I'm a bird watcher – have you ever seen a big blue veined throbber? (Advanced)

15. I'm the spokesman for a bicycle shop

16. I'm a male impersonator

17. I used to work at a bubble gum factory but I quit when my boss chewed me out

TALK ABOUT DATING...

Talk about dating...

1. This last girl I met on Match – I caught her lying – under some other guy

2. I stopped dating this one girl because she used too many 4-letter words – Stop! Don't! Quit That!

3. I had this one date who wanted me to treat her like royalty – so I took her to Burger King and Dairy Queen.

4. She wanted me to take her to this expensive restaurant, so I finally gave in and drove her there. Then she got mad because I didn't take her inside!

5. I started dating this anorexic girl but then I started seeing less and less of her

6. The last long distance relationship I had was telescopic

7. I found out how to seduce heavy girls – it's a piece of cake.

8. I dated a devout Buddhist once and never called her again. I ran into her one night while she was working at a pizza joint. Trying to ease the tension, I jokingly said, "Make me one with everything."

She charged me a hundred bucks. I asked her for the change. She told me "Change comes from within," and slammed the cash register shut.

9. I used to date this woman who was a mime, but I never could get close to her because I always felt there was some kind of wall between us.

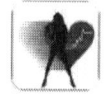

10. I once dated a woman who proposed... that we start seeing other people.

A LULL IN THE CONVERSATION?

A lull in the conversation

1. So, do you meet any attractive interesting men here besides me?

2. You can't have everything, where would you put it?

3. If it's zero degrees outside today, and it's supposed to be twice as cold tomorrow – how cold is it going to be?

4. This guy outside asked me for a dollar for a sandwich – I asked him to show me the sandwich first.

5. He said he hadn't eaten for 3 days – I told him I wish I had his willpower

6. This morning, I shot an elephant in my pajamas – how it got in my pajamas, I'll never know.

7. If I can't have access to your e-mail or phone number, how about your refrigerator?

8. You should see my collection of seashells – I have them scattered on beaches all over the world.

9. I stayed in a really old hotel the other night – they gave me a wakeup letter

10. I asked the lady at the front desk of the hotel if they have turndown service – She said sure – I wouldn't date you if you were the last guy on earth.

11. How do you know when you're out of invisible ink?

12. Have you ever wondered why the third hand on a watch is called a second hand?

13. (On the phone) if you can't hear me, it's because I'm in parentheses

14. Enough of me talking about myself – now why don't you talk about me.

15. I met my ex in a revolving door, and then we started going around together.

16. She was a great housekeeper – she got to keep the house.

17. Did you hear about the girl who rode her bicycle down a cobblestone street? She said I'll never come this way again.

18. Did you hear about the cannibal who passed his friend in the jungle?

19. Did you hear about the trapeze artist who was caught in the act?

20. Have you ever wondered if cannibals think clowns taste funny?

21. Did you hear about the two gay Irish judges who tried each other? One was Gerald Fitzpatrick and the other was Patrick Fitzgerald.

22. If you want a committed man, you should look in a mental hospital

23. They say a guy's not complete until he's married – then he's finished

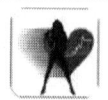

24. I can tell people are judgmental just by looking at them.

25. You can tell a lot by the way a woman walks. Like if she walks away, she's probably not into you.

26. The worst thing about being bipolar is that it's so awesome.

27. You can tell a lot about a woman by secretly reading her emails.

28. Have you ever wondered why Ms. Universe is always won by someone from earth?

29. Do you know what I like about you? You can't think of anything either?

30. I really like to tell you what a great job you're doing – But I just can't bring myself to it.

31. It's apparent to everyone around us how attracted you are to me, but you have to stop coming on so strong to me, because it's not working….

32. If I stole something, would you chase me?

33. Have you ever wondered who decides when the applause should die down? It's probably a group decision…

34. "I am," is the shortest sentence in the English Language – "I do," is the longest sentence…

35. There is no present – there's only the immediate future and the recent past

36. Always do whatever's next

37. When cheese gets its picture taken, what does it say?

39. Everywhere is within walking distance if you have the time…

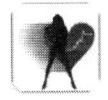

40. The last thing I remember was someone saying, "No need for alarm"

41. The surest way to remain a winner is to win once, then not play anymore…

42. Some people have become so used to the life they're living that they think it's normal.

43. We imprison all the petty thieves, but the real good ones are elected to office.

44. When I found out my toaster wasn't waterproof, I was shocked!

45. These new corduroy pillows are making headlines

46. When the 5-foot psychic escaped from jail there was a small medium at large

47. "What if Alexander Graham Bell's name were Alexander Graham Siren? The phone wouldn't ring, it would GO EERRRRRRRRRRRRRRRRR! (Make a noise like a siren)

48. If I had a dollar for every time I got distracted, I wish I had some ice cream…

49. Always do the right thing – it will gratify some and astonish others

Random responses

1. Those are my principles, and if you don't like them…well I have others.

2. A man does not control his own fate, a woman does that for him

3. I hate to see you go but I like to watch you leave

4. Whatever it is, I'm against it.

5. Marriage is a wonderful institution, but who wants to live in an institution

6. The secret of life is honesty and fair dealing. If you can fake that, you've got it made.

ADVANCED LINES TO ESCALATE (ONLY AFTER RAPPORT)

Advanced lines to escalate (only after rapport has been established)

Use the following lines only when you're sure she's into you and you're ready to escalate and transition into sex. I do not recommend these lines for opening or if you haven't yet established rapport.

1. You've been a bad girl, now go to my room

2. Congratulations! You've just won "the anonymous award" and the grand prize is a night with me!

3. Do you know, your hair and my pillow are perfectly color coordinated?

4. I wish you would keep your hands to myself

5. Would you like to have breakfast? Do you want me to pick you up at your place or just nudge you?

6. Do you like sitting up front, or do you like it in the rear?

7. Excuse me, but can you tell your breasts to stop staring at my eyes...

8. Can you touch your elbows behind your back?

9. I came over here to talk to you because I thought you were attractive – but now I'm not so sure. Let me look closer.

10. So do you like strawberries or blueberries? Why? Because I need to know what kind of pancakes to make you in the morning.

11. Have you ever slept with a stranger? I'm so glad we've been introduced

12. You've got curves and I don't have any brakes

13. Could I ask you for a small favor? I have a headache and I hear that sex is the best cure.

14. Bitches hate it when you're sexist.

15. YouTube Myspace and I'll Google your Yahoo

16. I like the way you're wearing that blouse, but honestly, I think it'd look better on the floor.

17. Do you work for UPS or Fedex? I could have sworn I saw you checking out my package.

18. You should surprise your roommate and not come home tonight

19. Does this smell like chloroform to you?

20. Have you ever tried a roofy?

21. Either way I'm going to have sex with you tonight so; you might as well be there with me

22. Sometimes I go bird watching.... Would you like to see a big blue veined throbber? I can show it to you.

23. I knew they should have never given women the vote.

24. A woman's place is in the kitchen and the bedroom – and the extent of her travels between the two....

25. I'll bet you I can kiss your lips without even touching you – close your eyes – (kiss her) then say, OK - you win...

26. Then say, I'll bet you ten dollars I can grab your boobs without even touching your blouse....

27. I think you should know what people are saying behind your back. She'll ask, what's that? They are saying that you have a nice ass

28. Do you have any (state your ethnic heritage, Hispanic, Asian, Irish etc.) in you? Would you like some? (You better be pretty drunk with this one)

29. Let me show you how I can speak English and French at the same time

30. That's a nice blouse – can I talk you out of it?

31. Every woman is beautiful – sometimes it just takes the right amount of alcohol to see it.

32. If you're feeling down, maybe I can feel you up.

33. You are so sexy when you start flirting with me like that (especially if she's doing nothing)

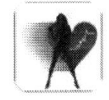

34. So, what parts of your body are the ones that get you turned on the most? You mean like right here, and like this? If she says, "I don't have any," you say, "Liar" and if she says, "I'm not telling you" – then you say it's usually right here (then touch the back of her neck)

35. Are those tic tacs in your blouse pocket or are you just happy to see me?

36. You like sleeping? Me too - Maybe we should try it together sometime...

This concludes the Appendix. Last but not least are my acknowledgements

ACKNOWLEDGEMENTS:

I would like to thank the following scientists, authors, dating experts, to all the girls I've loved before (not mentioned personally) and any others I forgot to mention who helped contribute to my education and awareness in the art and science of Love and Attraction.

	Azis	Ansari	Comedian, author of Modern Romance
Dr.	Scott	Barry Kaufman	Psychologist, author of Mating Intelligence Unleashed
Dr.	Joyce	Brothers	Psychologist and author of many books on love and attraction
Dr.	David	Buss	Evolutionary Psychologist, author of several books on Love and Attraction
	Jack	Canfield	Author of Chicken Soup for the Soul: True Love
	Jason	Capital	America's *1 Honest Dating Coach
Dr.	Steven	Covey	Bestselling author of 7 habits of highly effective people
	David	DeAngelo	Dating Expert, Best Selling Author of Double Your Dating
Dr.	Helen	Fisher	Anthropologist, Author of several books on Love and Attraction
Dr.	Glen	Geher	Psychologist, author of Mating Intelligence Unleashed
	Malcolm	Gladwell	Best Selling Author of Blink
Dr.	Sai	Goddam	Computer Scientist, author of A Billion Wicked

Dr.	Jeffrey	Hall	Communications Expert, author of The Five Flirting Styles
Dr.	Yuval	Harari	Historian, author of Sapiens
	Lance	Mason	Dating Expert
Dr.	Cindy	Meston	Psychologist, author of Why Women Have Sex
Dr.	Geoffrey	Miller	Evolutionary Psychologist, Author of several books on Love and Attraction
Dr.	Desmond	Morris	Zoologist, University of Oxford, Author of The Naked Ape
Dr.	Ogi	Ogas	Neuroscientist, Author of A Billion Wicked Thoughts
	Tony	Robbins	Motivational speaker and relationship expert and Best Selling Author
	David	Wygant	Dating Expert
	Neil	Strauss	Dating Expert, Author of "The Game"

The End

This has been How to Attract Women, Irresistible Humor and Body Language Secrets

Written and narrated by Leonardo Bustos, Copyright 2015,

Printed in Great Britain
by Amazon